Global Culture and Sport Series

Series edited by **Stephen Wagg**, Professor, Leeds Beckett University, UK and **David Andrews**, Professor & Director of Graduate Studies, University of Maryland School of Public Health, USA

Titles include:

Emmanuelle Tulle and Cassandra Phoenix (*editors*)
PHYSICAL ACTIVITY AND SPORT IN LATER LIFE
Critical Perspectives

Alex Channon and Christopher R. Matthews
GLOBAL PERSPECTIVES ON WOMEN IN COMBAT SPORTS
Women Warriors Around the World

Stephen Wagg
THE LONDON OLYMPICS OF 2012
Politics, Promises and Legacies

Tendai Chari and Nhamo A. Mhiripiri (*editors*)
AFRICAN FOOTBAL, IDENTITY POLITICS AND GLOBAL MEDIA NARRATIVES
The Legacy of the FIFA2010 World Cup

Jesper Andreasson and Thomas Johansson
THE GLOBAL GYM
Gender, Health and Pedagogies

Chuka Onwumechili and Gerard Akindes (*editors*)
IDENTITY AND NATION IN AFRICAN FOOTBALL
Fans, Community and Clubs

Nico Schulenkorf and Daryl Adair (*editors*)
GLOBAL SPORT-FOR-DEVELOPMENT
Critical Perspectives

Alejandro Quiroga
FOOTBALL AND NATIONAL IDENTITIES IN SPAIN

John Karamichas
THE OLYMPIC GAMES AND THE ENVIRONMENT

Aaron Beacom
INTERNATIONAL DIPLOMACY AND THE OLYMPIC MOVEMENT
The New Mediators

Dikaia Chatziefstathiou and Ian P. Henry
DISCOURSES OF OLYMPISM
From the Sorbonne 1894 to London 2012

Mike Dennis and Jonathan Grix
SPORT UNDER COMMUNISM
Behind the East German 'Miracle'

Mahfoud Amara
SPORT, POLITICS AND SOCIETY IN THE ARAB WORLD

Graeme Hayes and John Karamichas (*editors*)
OLYMPIC GAMES, MEGA-EVENTS AND CIVIL SOCIETIES

Peter Millward
THE GLOBAL FOOTBALL LEAGUE

Holly Thorpe
SNOWBOARDING BODIES IN THEORY AND PRACTICE

Jonathan Long and Karl Spacklen (*editors*)
SPORT AND CHALLENGES TO RACISM

John Harris
RUGBY UNION AND GLOBALIZATION
An Odd-Shaped World

Pirkko Markula (*editor*)
OLYMPIC WOMEN AND THE MEDIA
International Perspectives

Roger Levermore and Aaron Beacom (*editors*)
SPORT AND INTERNATIONAL DEVELOPMENT

Global Culture and Sport Series
Series Standing Order ISBN 9780-2-305-7818-0 (Hardback)
(*Outside North America only*)

You can receive future titles in this series as they are published by placing a standing order. Please contact your bookseller or, in case of difficulty, write to us at the address below with your name and address, the title of the series and the ISBNs quoted above.

Customer Services Department, Macmillan Distribution Ltd, Houndmills, Basingstoke, Hampshire RG21 6XS, England

Physical Activity and Sport in Later Life
Critical Perspectives

Edited by

Emmanuelle Tulle
Glasgow Caledonian University, UK

and

Cassandra Phoenix
University of Exeter, UK

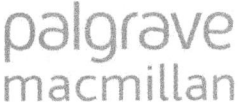

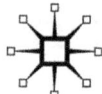

Selection, introduction and editorial matter © Emmanuelle Tulle and Cassandra Phoenix 2015
Remaining chapters © Contributors 2015
All rights reserved. No reproduction, copy or transmission of this publication may be made without written permission.

No portion of this publication may be reproduced, copied or transmitted save with written permission or in accordance with the provisions of the Copyright, Designs and Patents Act 1988, or under the terms of any licence permitting limited copying issued by the Copyright Licensing Agency, Saffron House, 6–10 Kirby Street, London EC1N 8TS.

Any person who does any unauthorized act in relation to this publication may be liable to criminal prosecution and civil claims for damages.

The authors have asserted their rights to be identified as the authors of this work in accordance with the Copyright, Designs and Patents Act 1988.

First published 2015 by
PALGRAVE MACMILLAN

Palgrave Macmillan in the UK is an imprint of Macmillan Publishers Limited, registered in England, company number 785998, of Houndmills, Basingstoke, Hampshire RG21 6XS.

Palgrave Macmillan in the US is a division of St Martin's Press LLC, 175 Fifth Avenue, New York, NY 10010.

Palgrave Macmillan is the global academic imprint of the above companies and has companies and representatives throughout the world.

Palgrave® and Macmillan® are registered trademarks in the United States, the United Kingdom, Europe and other countries.

ISBN: 978–1–137–42931–5

This book is printed on paper suitable for recycling and made from fully managed and sustained forest sources. Logging, pulping and manufacturing processes are expected to conform to the environmental regulations of the country of origin.

A catalogue record for this book is available from the British Library.

Library of Congress Cataloging-in-Publication Data
   Physical activity and sport in later life : critical perspectives / Emmanuelle Tulle, Glasgow Caledonian University, UK, Cassandra Phoenix, University of Exeter, UK.
   pages cm
   ISBN 978–1–137–42931–5
   1. Physical fitness for older people. 2. Sports for older people. 3. Exercise for older people. 4. Aging—Physiological aspects. I. Tulle, Emmanuelle. II. Phoenix, Cassandra.
GV482.6.P48 2015
613.7′0446—dc23   2015019258

Contents

Notes on Contributors	vii
1 Introduction: Rethinking Physical Activity and Sport in Later Life *Emmanuelle Tulle and Cassandra Phoenix*	1
2 Physical Activity and Sedentary Behaviour: A Vital Politics of Old Age? *Emmanuelle Tulle*	9
3 Physical Activity and Narratives of Successful Ageing *Elizabeth C. J. Pike*	21
4 Fitness and Consumerism in Later Life *Paul Higgs and Chris Gilleard*	32
5 Type 2 Diabetes and Commitment of Seniors to Adapted Physical Activity within the French System of Therapeutic Education *Nathalie Barth and Claire Perrin*	43
6 Pathways to Masters Sport: Sharing Stories from Sport 'Continuers', 'Rekindlers' and 'Late Bloomers' *Rylee A. Dionigi*	54
7 Keeping It in the Family: The Generational Transmission of Physical Activity *Victoria J. Palmer*	69
8 Physical Activity Programmes in Residential Care Settings *Mary-Ann Kluge*	81
9 Physical Activity and Dementia: Tai Chi as Narrative Care *Gary Kenyon*	92
10 The Multidimensionality of Pleasure in Later Life Physical Activity *Cassandra Phoenix and Noreen Orr*	101
11 The Contingencies of Exercise Science in a Globalising World: Ageing Chinese Canadians and their Play and Pleasure in Exercise *Shannon Jette and Patricia Vertinsky*	113

12 Fell Running in Later Life: Irresponsible Intoxication or
   Existential Capital? 124
   Sarah Nettleton

13 Ageing and Embodied Masculinities in Physical Activity
   Settings: From Flesh to Theory and Back Again 137
   Andrew C. Sparkes

14 Ageing Women Still Play Games: (Auto)ethnographic
   Research in a Fitness Intervention 149
   Gertrud Pfister and Verena Lenneis

15 Physical Activity among Older Adults with Visual
   Impairment: Considerations for Ageing Well with Sight Loss 161
   Meridith Griffin

16 Local Environments and Activity in Later Life: Meaningful
   Experiences in Green and Blue Spaces 175
   Sarah L. Bell and Benedict W. Wheeler

Index 187

Notes on Contributors

Nathalie Barth holds a PhD from the Université Claude Bernard Lyon 1, France, where she is a teaching assistant and researcher. She is the author of publications on the sociology of sport and health, notably on adapted physical activity, commitment and empowerment of people with chronic illness (*Leisure and Society*, 2014).

Sarah L. Bell is an associate research fellow at the European Centre for Environment and Human Health, University of Exeter, UK. She is interested in developing mixed method and interdisciplinary approaches to explore the complex interrelations between lived environments and human wellbeing. Sarah's recent work on the development of GPS and geo-narrative approaches has been published in *Area* (DOI: 10.1111/area.12152).

Rylee A. Dionigi is an associate professor at the School of Human Movement Studies at Charles Sturt University, Bathurst, NSW, Australia. She has published in the fields of sport sociology, ageing and physical activity, exercise psychology and leisure studies.

Chris Gilleard is a visiting research fellow in the Division of Psychiatry at UCL, UK. He is co-author with Paul Higgs of *Ageing, Corporeality and Embodiment* (2013).

Meridith Griffin is an assistant professor in the Department of Health, Aging and Society at McMaster University, Ontario, Canada. Her research encompasses a number of topic areas, including ageing, health and wellbeing, disability, gender and embodiment – particularly as these play out in the social and cultural realms of leisure and physical activity.

Paul Higgs is Professor of Sociology of Ageing in the Division of Psychiatry at UCL, UK. He is co-author with Chris Gilleard of *Rethinking Old Age: Theorising the Fourth Age* (2015). He is co-investigator on two ESRC/NIHR dementia research programmes and is a fellow of both the Academy of Social Sciences and the Gerontological Society of America.

Shannon Jette is an assistant professor in the Department of Kinesiology at the University of Maryland, USA. Her research focuses on the critical sociological analysis of women's health across the lifespan, and has been published in such journals as *Health, Risk & Society* and *Sport, Education & Society*.

Gary Kenyon is Professor and Chair, Gerontology Department, St. Thomas University, Fredericton, New Brunswick, Canada. He is co-editor (with Ernst Bohlmeijer and William L. Randall) of *Storying Later Life* and co-editor of a Special Issue of the *Journal of Aging Studies*. His main research interests are in narrative gerontology and narrative care.

Mary-Ann Kluge is Professor of Health Sciences at the University of Colorado, Colorado Springs (UCCS), USA, whose work focuses on older adult fitness, wellness, and sports participation. She is Director of the Center for Active Living at an Integrated Healthcare Services Center. Her research, writing and public speaking is primarily on how to best support older adults' discovery and continuation of a 'physically active self' through the lifecourse.

Verena Lenneis is a PhD student in the Department of Nutrition, Exercise and Sports at the University of Copenhagen, Denmark. Her research focus lies in the field of sport sociology and gender studies.

Sarah Nettleton is Professor of Sociology in the Department of Sociology at the University of York, UK. She is the author of *Sociology of Health and Illness* (2013), third edition, and has also published on health, illness and embodiment.

Noreen Orr is an associate research fellow at the University of Exeter Medical School's European Centre for Environment and Human Health. Her research focuses upon how older adults create and manage distinctive later life identities; the impact of ageing on health and well-being; and the ageing body within the natural environment.

Victoria J. Palmer is a PhD student at Glasgow Caledonian University, UK, and a researcher at the Universities of Glasgow and Edinburgh. Her PhD work is a close examination of physical activity practices and beliefs within three-generational families, drawing on sociological and sports science insights.

Claire Perrin is Associate Professor of Sociology at the Université Claude Bernard Lyon 1, France. She is the editor of *Corps et témoignage* and author of works on the sociologies of adapted physical activity, the body, chronic illness and health.

Gertrud Pfister is a professor in the Department of Nutrition, Exercise and Sports at the University of Copenhagen, Denmark. She has PhDs in Sociology and History as well as two honorary doctorates. In the past 30 years she has conducted research and published widely in the history of sport and sport sociology. She is currently a member of the executive board of Women Sport International.

Cassandra Phoenix is Senior Lecturer in Qualitative Health Research at the University of Exeter Medical School's European Centre for Environment and Human Health, UK. Her work draws upon the sociology of ageing, the body and physical culture. She was primary investigator for the ESRC funded 'Moving Stories' project, which examined the role of physical activity in shaping expectations and experiences of ageing (Ref ES/I009779/1).

Elizabeth Pike is Head of Sport Development and Management, Reader in Sociology of Sport and Exercise, Chair of the Anita White Foundation at the University of Chichester, UK. She is co-editor (with Simon Beames) of *Sports in Society: Issues and Controversies* and *Outdoor Adventure and Social Theory* (2013). She is president of the International Sociology of Sport Association.

Andrew C. Sparkes is Professor of Sport, Physical Activity and Leisure at Leeds Beckett University, UK. He is co-author (with Brett Smith) of *Qualitative Research Methods in Sport, Exercise and Health: From Process to Product* (2014), and co-editor (with Maggie O'Neill and Brian Roberts) of *Advances in Biographical Methods: Creative Applications* (2015). Andrew's work is nomadic in nature, operating in the cracks between disciplinary boundaries.

Emmanuelle Tulle is Reader in Sociology at Glasgow Caledonian University, UK. She is the author of *Ageing, the Body and Social Change: Running in Later Life* (Palgrave Macmillan, 2008) and other publications on the sociologies of old age, sport and physical activity and the body.

Patricia Vertinsky is Distinguished University Scholar and Professor of Kinesiology at the University of British Columbia in Vancouver, Canada. She is the co-editor (with Jennifer Hargreaves) of *Physical Culture, Power and the Body* (2006) and other publications on the history and sociology of physical culture, exercise and sport.

Benedict W. Wheeler is a senior research fellow at the University of Exeter Medical School's European Centre for Environment and Human Health, UK. He is a health geographer with a range of publications on the interconnections between environment, health and health inequalities, such as 'Does living by the coast improve health and wellbeing?' (*Health & Place*, 2012).

1
Introduction: Rethinking Physical Activity and Sport in Later Life
Emmanuelle Tulle and Cassandra Phoenix

Introduction

Becoming and being old is not what it used to be! How we imagined people and ourselves would grow old has been undergoing significant transformations. Babies born today can expect to live very long lives – well into their 80s – at least in the affluent West. Those we refer to as babyboomers (a birth cohort spanning the end of World War II and the early 1960s) are already pioneering long living, and their parents haven't done too badly either. This is quite a remarkable demographic transformation, one that has received plenty of policy, press and academic attention, not all of it very positive.

For the last 50 years, the social sciences have been mapping the wider context in which we are ageing and, of critical importance, the resources – cultural, symbolic and practical – we have been harnessing to make sense of this extraordinary phenomenon. What has been exposed in this scholarship is a tension, a fracture even, between how people actually *live* their lives and theories of ageing. On the one hand, we can point to long lives as opening up opportunities for imagining new ways of organising and punctuating lives and more generally individual futures. On the other hand, it has also been shown that we are still hampered by modes of thought which have their roots in deterministic, reductionist and ultimately negative conceptions of the ageing process. Sometimes this fracture can be seen in scholarly endeavours and is often indistinguishable from what separates particular disciplines. We contend that it is present in the area of sport and physical activity, particularly manifested in the divide between the life sciences and the social sciences.

This is not immediately visible however. Indeed, there seems to be consensus across various areas of social and academic life that physical activity is a good thing. Its physiological benefits have been well reported in the life sciences and its psychological benefits appear undeniable. The message has extended to the old with the emergence since the 1990s of evidence demonstrating how physical activity is a good way to prevent (or at any rate slow down) many of the conditions still associated with ageing and old age, for example, sarcopenia, cancers, cardiovascular and respiratory diseases and a raft of late onset conditions such as Type 2 diabetes. Policy-makers at all levels of government have been convinced of the need to promote physical activity amongst older people. Moreover, particular responsibility has been devolved to care providers to design strategies for improving participation rates among this population group which continue to have lower levels of physical activity than the rest of the population. As has been demonstrated elsewhere, social and cultural change has transformed late life experiences, a process to which older people have actively contributed by engaging in consumption, new forms of leisure and by not accepting physical decline or marginalisation as a fact of life. However, when it comes to physical activity, older people have been more reticent to align to new norms of participation, as the statistics on physical activity participation demonstrate, and this contributes to the decline of their ageing body.

Reference is often made to Hippocrates, Galen and other Ancient Greeks recommending the incorporation of physical activity into one's life regimen to give legitimacy to what elsewhere has been termed the turn to physical activity. There is plentiful evidence that, over time, physical activity recommendations have been inflected by class, gender, age and race norms of appropriate physicality. Although our forebears did not have access to all the labour saving technologies which contribute to increases in inactivity, their embodiment was heavily regulated and cannot be used as a model for how we think about contemporary approaches to physical exertion. And yet, the past is often held up, especially in the biomedical sciences, as the golden age of lifelong physical activity.

We are therefore concerned that the complexities and subtleties which affect whether and how we use our bodies as we become older have been overlooked. For instance, women, people from minority ethnic groups, people of lower socio-economic status and disabled older adults are particularly prone to inactivity, and this goes hand in hand with poor health and frailty. This scenario raises a number of questions. Specifically, how can we now convince different groups of older people that they should be more physically active, that it will be worth the effort, that it will lead to significant improvements in their health and mobility? How do we persuade them that it is a feasible prospect? What are the personal, *physical* and cultural barriers to people being receptive to the health messages permeating the constant encouragement of certain older adults to shift their disposition away from a preference to 'take it easy' toward an urge to be physically active on a regular basis? How do the various groups of older people who engage in physical activity experience it? What benefits are derived and do they reflect the benefits promoted in 'official' health messages? What can we learn from these experiences without setting impossible standards, which would doom to failure those who couldn't possibly match them? More to the point, what does the almost frenetic noise around trying to find ways of coaxing the old out of their chairs and to a gym hall or the outdoors tell us about contemporary ageing? Does it represent a challenge to normative instructions on how to age appropriately? Pursuing questions such as these has the potential to move our understanding of later life sport and physical activity beyond its common framing as *only* a (prescribed) 'solution' to the 'problems' of old age.

We are mindful that much research within this framework is given legitimacy by the deployment of largely alarmist statements about population ageing and the anticipated ill-health burden it will impose on already stretched public finances. While we do not take issue with the fact of population ageing, we are concerned that this mantra can be used to promote knowledge and new forms of interventions that might raise inflated hopes about the potential of physical activity and sport to alleviate the bodily changes associated with physiological ageing. For example, there are older adults who appear to fulfil and in some cases even exceed physical activity recommendations: the very fit and participants in the Masters movement. It would be easy to see these people as models of 'good ageing' for others to emulate. However, as eloquently demonstrated by a number of contributors to this collection, while it is important to identify what lessons might be learned from these people's experiences, care must be taken not to fall into the trap of positioning them as heroes of ageing. Likewise, we must remain aware of the ease with which physical activity can be seen as an anti-ageing practice. In other words, we should consider its impact on the extent to which we view old age as a legitimate part of living that has meaning and value in its own right. At stake here is the relegation of those whose bodies have lost almost all function to the margins of society, reinforcing the separation between a third age of activity and agelessness and a fourth age of frailty, dependency and confinement to medicalised institutions.

It is precisely these concerns that have prompted us to devise this collection and to invite social scientists committed to extending this field to contribute their insights. Through the pages that follow, we aspire to meet two broad objectives: first, to provide readers with expert conceptual analyses of how physical activity and sport in later life is socially, historically and culturally located and second, to bring these conceptual analyses to life through state of the art, critically informed, empirical research. Our contributors originate from a number of disciplines (including sociology, social gerontology, sport science, physical cultural studies, health geography, psychology) and share a range of principles. Specifically, some contributors prioritised the voices and experiences of older people and sought to understand how older people ascribe meaning and value to what they are (or are not) doing. This involves situating concerns with ageing and old age in a rich context – one that exceeds the traditional boundaries of physical activity and sport – to understand how our growing acceptance that older people *should* be physically active has arisen and developed. It also requires consideration of the potential opportunities and barriers that might impact upon the achievement of the aim to encourage older adults to be less sedentary alongside older adults' own aspirations to 'control' their lives in ways that facilitate acceptable levels of satisfaction and dignity. Thus other contributors gave critical focus to the societal context in which physical activity is promoted.

We hope that this collection will make an important contribution to scholarship by encouraging readers to think critically about the role that physical activity and sport can play in how we age while initiating dialogues regarding creative solutions to what are increasingly perceived as 'problems': the low levels of physical activity amongst the old, and indeed the old themselves. Our 15 contributions to this edited collection address the question of physical activity in later life from different angles, disciplinary backgrounds and with different groups of older people. We have organised them by themes, which are outlined below. That said, it is worth noting that each contribution exceeds its central theme by dealing with a wealth of issues, providing rich illustrations and presenting rigorous interpretations. We invite readers to read all or most of these chapters to appreciate the subtleties of the arguments presented in each.

The first three contributions replace the question of physical activity within its discursive and cultural context. These chapters are scene-setters: they identify the key characteristics of neoliberal societies and how these affect how ageing is imagined. They take issue with the increasing tendency to exhort people to become physically activity as the norm of 'ageing well' and to demonise those who do not comply with these physical activity exhortations.

The collection proceeds with Tulle (Chapter 2) who locates discussions of physical activity in their wider discursive context. She develops a critical examination of the extension to be physically active to that of avoiding being sedentary. Thus sitting down has become a new public health emergency, and she sees this as a manifestation of the increasing tendency to control lives and our bodies, an extension of government. Pike (Chapter 3) engages in a critical analysis of how physical activity has been held up as the solution to biological decline and reconstructed as a 'successful ageing' strategy. Using a range of documentary sources, she shows how the responsibility for ageing well has shifted from the state to an individual level. Gilleard and Higgs (Chapter 4) show how physical activity has emerged as a constituent of consumer culture and is used as a way of enticing people to view a fit and active old age as a good old age. They reflect on the association between physical activity, fitness and health, which can lead those who do not fulfil physical activity requirements to be reconstructed as having failed. They also caution readers on the limits of physical activity as the solution to physical decline. By taking a strong critical stance, these 3 chapters provide the backdrop against which we can begin to imagine alternative approaches to physical activity and the opportunities and challenges that they themselves might pose.

The next theme deals with the process of becoming physically active. Chapters 5, 6 and 7 bring to light the complexities, vulnerabilities but also time-bound nature of physical activity and sporting careers. Barth and Perrin (Chapter 5) focus their investigation on patients with late onset diabetes (Type 2 Diabetes). These patients' experiences are full of valuable lessons for how to enable the transition from physical activity as medical prescription to physical activity as a self-determined practice in later life. Thus they use the concept of *career* to make sense of the pathways and the different stages which might lead to an orientation to the body that is no longer strictly medicalised. Dionigi (Chapter 6) proposes a typology of engagement with Masters sports – continuers, rekindlers and late bloomers – to show that maintaining an exercise practise takes commitment, can be easily disrupted but if re-started can lead to renewed engagement and enjoyment. Palmer (Chapter 7) focuses on the role played by *family* in facilitating a physical activity career. What makes her work distinctive is that she highlights something which, recast in the discourse of decline, is not intuitive: the central role that grandparents play in the creation and reproduction of family cultures of physical activity.

The next theme which our collection addresses is the role that care settings (and the philosophies of care which are used to run them) can play in hindering or initiating alternative understandings of physical activity which can lead to richer lives during deep old age. Kluge's contribution (Chapter 8) describes an innovative programme of leisure and physical activities in a residential care retirement community. The programme was co-created by residents, residential care staff and university partners with the aim of providing activities that responded to people's needs, values, goals and preferences while fostering a sense of autonomy. Thus, the purpose of physical activity in this setting was not reduced to physical outcome measures alone (such as improvements in physical function), but rather to promote engagement in community life. Interestingly, Kluge then reflects on the consequences of selling the residential facility to another company which took the decision to discontinue this innovative programme. In Chapter 9, Kenyon describes how he uses Tai Chi to accompany people with dementia in the negotiation of what he terms 'thicker' narratives of care. Tai Chi is used to recover and retell people's stories through movement rather than as part of a programme which prioritises adherence to strict performance objectives. Kenyon's approach brings to the foreground the potential of physical engagement to enrich people's lives by reconnecting them to their apparently lost selves while also evoking feelings of pleasure.

Pleasure is a theme that spans Chapters 10, 11 and 12. Phoenix and Orr (Chapter 10) stumbled on the theme of pleasure in their study of physically active older adults. They noted an absent discussion of pleasure in the literature that addresses late life physicality in relation to ageing well. Armed with an unplanned wealth of data on pleasure, which drew attention to different ways of enjoying movement, they were able to construct a typology of pleasure and reflect on the implications of this finding for practice. Meanwhile, Jette and Vertinsky (Chapter 11) highlight how their analysis of interviews with Chinese-Canadian women unveiled innovative and creative approaches to physical engagement that combined Traditional Chinese Medicine and Western approaches to health and medicine to devise ways of moving the body. Movement in this context was not in the calculated pursuit of health and the management of functional decline as dictated by external agencies, but in the pursuit of happiness and life balance. Nettleton (Chapter 12) also describes participants who want to be in charge of how they use their bodies: fell runners. She shows that older fell runners are compelled to continue engaging in an activity which is potentially dangerous because they have, over the years, become intoxicated with the pleasures of running, to the extent that running is not something that they ought to do but something that they viscerally need to do, for reasons other than health.

Sparkes as well as Pfister and Linneis address our penultimate theme, gender, in Chapters 13 and 14. They approach gender from apparently different directions, but one concern unites them: self-making/re-storying and the ageing body. They both produce highly personal but also sociologically pertinent accounts using auto-ethnography. Sparkes (Chapter 13) explores the potential threat to his masculinity that his changing physical capabilities might pose. He eschews the decline narrative, which others have already found hinders how we can retain meaning as we age and in the search for other, more satisfying ways of narrating his own relationship to his body, appeals to ways of narrating the body and self which do not trap him in a sterile choice between rejecting decline and failing to embrace what his body can still accomplish. Meanwhile, Pfister and Lenneis (Chapter 14) offer a critique of the enfeeblement of ageing women. They describe an encounter with female participants involved in an intervention designed to measure the physiological impact of participating in the team sport of floorball. Pfister joined the women in their socialisation into the sport and their discovery not only that they could become good at floorball in older age, but also enjoy it on a range of different levels.

These gendered experiences draw attention to the crucial role played by structures in influencing what people can accomplish as they age. The transformative power of physical activity cannot be envisaged without raising fundamental but also personal questions about the best way to become old and deal with the question of physical change and presence in the physical world. These questions have particular pertinence and resonance for the people whose experiences inform the final theme of the collection: place and space. We chose to close the collection with this theme because it takes us back to our original problematisation of physical activity: it cannot be seen first and foremost as a problem of motivation or individual responsibility. Some people will find their ability to be physically active significantly curtailed or indeed supported by their physical environment.

Griffin's chapter (Chapter 15) draws from the experiences of older people with sight loss. She describes the barriers to physical activity that can be a consequence of visual impairment, especially when sight loss intersects with other medical conditions. She shows the practical challenges that these people face in accessing (physically and emotionally) spaces and places that facilitate the enjoyment and pleasures that our other contributors have argued can result from meaningful forms of physical activity. Using an approach informed by the social model of disability, Griffin shows that the higher risk of exclusion of older people with impairments from physical activity opportunities can have a negative impact on their psycho-emotional well-being. Bell and Wheeler's contribution (Chapter 16) also deals with well-being and its connection to the natural environment. Using the innovative method of *geo-narratives* they show that people value green (countryside) and blue (coastal) spaces as places in which they can share meaningful experiences with others. While physical decrements might put some spaces out of bounds, the presence of other, easier to negotiate spaces enables older people to maintain a presence in the world through their physical selves. This research reinforces the message that there is more to the purpose of physical activity in later life than a retreat to the body as *the* object of intervention.

2
Physical Activity and Sedentary Behaviour: A Vital Politics of Old Age?
Emmanuelle Tulle

Introduction

A few years ago I wrote an article about physical activity and the positioning of sports science in the anti-ageing project (Tulle, 2008a). As I argued then, a particular narrative pervaded the sport science literature which contributed to the reconstruction of ageing bodies as malleable and fit bodies. I questioned whether and how this narrative could open the way for a significant reconfiguration of old age, one which would begin to address the negative symbolic capital associated with ageing, when the science itself was steeped in the neoliberal project of promoting physical activity as a solution to the 'burden of ageing'. I concluded that it would be dangerous to accept the turn to physical activity as resistance to cultural marginalisation. Indeed what needs to be done first and foremost is to change the terms of the debates, to unsettle its discursive and ideological anchor. In addition, faced with the ambiguity of the scientific evidence and the apparent reluctance of a majority of older people to fulfil physical activity recommendations, rather than reject the prospect that physical activity could become an integral element of older people's lives, I proposed that it might be more fruitful to reframe it as a creative or pleasurable engagement with movement, rather than as health-related and anti-ageing behaviour.

Six years on it has become evident that the regulatory potential of physical activity has not dissipated. On the contrary, it appears to have strengthened with the discovery of sedentary behaviour as a determinant of ill-health and secondary ageing. An important feature of sedentary behaviour is that it is not the obverse of physical activity, but a separate problem in its own right with effects on health which are independent of physical activity (Owen et al., 2010). Put another way, one can fulfil the World Health Organisation Physical Activity recommendations but still be categorised as sedentary: the Active Couch Potato (Hamilton et al., 2008). This development is worthy of critical attention.

The turn to sedentary behaviour in the sport science and medicine literature appears to justify a corresponding urge to intervene in the lives of older people which, outside of institutions, could be construed as overly intrusive and a reinforcement of biopower (Peterson and Bunton, 1997). Therefore, in what follows I will (a) present a discursive analysis of recent sport science literature to chart the ways in which sedentariness has started to inflect concerns with physical activity, (b) map the constituent characteristics of this discursive expansion and (c) reflect on the glaring omissions in the design of interventions: an awareness of the internal conversation which older people engage in when they make decisions about the conduct of their everyday lives. Ultimately I will argue that the 'discovery' and inclusion of sedentary behaviour into a group relation with physical activity represents a key weapon in the prosecution of a 'vital politics' (Rose, 2007). This vital politics targets not simply the continuation of life, but the achievement of particular norms of living. Thus a version of agency as first and foremost bio-ethical is privileged.

The correct use of the body

The turn to physical activity (PA) in later life is part of a bigger project to encourage what Foucault (1997: 152) called 'the correct use of the body'. Foucault defined physical exercise as 'that technique by which one imposes on the body tasks that are both repetitive and different, but always graduated' (161). This is a timebound process which yields docile bodies and subjectification and through which power can be exercised without limit or end. PA can therefore be understood as a microphysics of power designed to map the individual body so that it can be better known and controlled as well as a macrophysics of power exercised on populations.

In previous work, I showed that this nexus (mapping, knowing and control) operated in different ways, corresponding to different modalities of behaviour and expectations. For instance, in Masters sport (Tulle, 2008b), the entire life of the athlete is given over to training. The athlete's life is split into segments made up of days, weeks, months and years, each populated by activities designed to enhance or maintain athletic capital.

This partitioning of the athlete's life has a multiplying effect as each segment feeds into a momentum driving towards a culmination. They are in effect dynamic, mutually reinforcing and functionally necessary building blocks. Both the body and the life of the athlete are literally reconfigured, instrumentalised and subjected to constant monitoring in the search for performance.

In Tulle (2008a) I observed this process of mapping, knowing and control nexus in the literature on PA in later life. The urge to promote PA as a norm of living in old age drove scientists, in their search for evidence that PA is a good thing for older adults, to apply this nexus to the depths of the body, in its physiological and cellular materiality. Whilst Masters athletes are in control of their disciplining, inactive older people emerge as largely passive and unknowing, subjected to exercise repetitions, the purpose of which is to yield better health outcomes, that is to say, significant musculo-skeletal, physiological and cellular reconfigurations. Thus engaging in PA for health is the acceptance of this nexus of regulation which, until recently, entailed only a partial reorganisation of life. The design of adapted, age-appropriate PA programmes manifested in official PA recommendations included specifying what proportion of life should be given over to exercise. In other words, how many segments should be set aside and how they should be used, but these segments were largely discrete divisions.

The discovery of the 'problem' of sedentary behaviour (SB) as a major health risk potentially subjects the *whole* life and the *whole* person to the mapping, knowing and control nexus. Indeed, as we will see later in this chapter, the problematisation of being inactive (and more precisely sitting) as a health-related behaviour with its own name and nosographic existence has also affected how sedentary subjects are created. It will also have implications for how the problem itself can be resolved, thereby placing not only the life, but also the soul of the 'sedentary' person under scrutiny. In fact, it could be argued that the turn to PA and now to SB is a key site in the application of a 'vital politics' (Rose, 2007).

Foucault's insights on exercise were written in the context of punishment. He was interested primarily in the embodiment of power, in the flesh and in the soul, in institutions. The turn to PA and SB is largely concerned with the transformation of bodies and volition, both inside and outside institutional settings, caught up in what Estes (1979) called the 'aging enterprise'. That is, the targets of markets and neoliberal forces. Thus, to better capture how SB, in the twenty-first century, operates as part of the apparatus of regulation, driven by the health imperative, I now turn to Rose's (1999, 2007) analysis of neoliberal regulation.

The attainment of the correct body

Contemporary life is characterised by new and very powerful forms of control over our conduct which are designed to 'instill...prudent relations to the self as the condition for liberty' (Rose, 1999: 243). This transformation of conduct towards prudence is inscribed in what Rose terms a 'vital politics'. Rose defines this as 'our growing capacities to control, manage, engineer, reshape and modulate the very vital capacities of human beings as living creatures' (2007: 3), which gives rise to an emergent form of life, enabled by five mutation pathways: (1) Molecularisation, (2) Optimisation, (3) Subjectification, (4) Somatic expertise and (5) Economies of vitality. What specifically is at stake here is the changed relationship to our bodies characterised by a distancing from, and thus objectification of, our bodies so that we can judge them and enhance them, making ourselves better than we are. This process is mediated, that is to say facilitated and produced, by a complex but ultimately market-led apparatus.

It could be argued that what distinguishes Foucault's insights from Rose's, and therefore liberal from neoliberal regulation, is the move beyond the correct use of the body to the *attainment* of the correct body itself, in the exercise of what Rose (2007) calls 'biological citizenship'. Another key element of vital politics and biological citizenship is the expectation that the individual will take an actuarial and future-oriented stance towards the control of his or her body, intervening now to prevent future decrements. This would not be possible without a fundamental shift in biology itself, from its status as a discipline originally tasked with the 'fathoming [and codifying] of nature's inner workings to a science which promises the re-engineering of the building blocks of life itself' (Fuller, 2011: 16).

In sum, I am positioning the turn to PA and its apparent expansion to SB as a manifestation of disciplinary power focused not only on the body (biopower) (Petersen and Bunton, 1997), but also on the soul and volition. The target of power is the individual who is to develop a Cartesian relationship to his/her body, accepting the health imperative as his/her chosen driving force. SB itself has attained an existence in its own right, that is it has ontological status which opens the way for the public scrutiny of everyday life, sanctioned by neoliberal forms of government.

Questions of behaviour and lifestyle changes are therefore brought to the fore as evidence (presented and analysed later in the chapter) mounts showing that people become more inactive with increasing age, and thus the success of interventions to change behaviour is certainly not assured. Whether we interpret this behavioural response to ageing as non-compliance, as resistance or as normative enfeeblement depends on our theoretical approach to agency.

Reflections on agency

As Katz (2013) has recently argued, in the field of health we tend to rely on the concept of lifestyle to talk about behaviours and in particular behaviour change. The determinants of our lifestyles are largely attributed to individual traits, which facilitate or hinder the adoption of health-appropriate behaviours. Katz shows that the focus on individuals as responsible for the acquisition of better lifestyles masks the latter's origins in social structures. He gives the example of falls, identified as a significant public health issue in later life. Fall interventions target individuals and their behaviours, aiming to accomplish lifestyle change, ignoring the gender and class basis of our actions, as well as the environmental, physical and policy barriers to behaviour change.

Archer (2003) could be used to complement Katz's critique. For Archer agency is indeed conditioned by structure and should be seen as the result of a process of deliberation which takes place in what she terms an 'internal conversation'. This process of deliberation cannot be reduced to rational choice or perceptual processes. She views the internal conversation as a manifestation of self-reflexivity and awareness of society which is unseen by the outsider. Our deliberative capacities are the bridge between structure and agency. They have causal efficacy because it is in these periods that individuals take stock of, and activate constraints or enablement to, action, as they find them and as they impinge on their lives. The notion of impingement is potentially interesting. For the American philosopher Harry Frankfurt (2004), what engages our deliberative capacities, that is, what drives us to do things, is not exclusively normative, via moral reasoning, rather it is what we care about, what matters to us. We might be confronted to conflicting forces and desires (to exercise for health *versus* the fear to engage in anything too strenuous), but the ultimate course of action will be informed by the knowledge we have of ourselves, our experiences of the world and ultimately what matters most to us (nervousness about exercising overriding the acceptance of the positive, yet deferred, benefits of a programme of exercise). A lifestyle change therefore can only take place as a result of the internal conversation which itself takes place at the intersection of societal pressures and individual habits, desires and, crucially, lifelong experiences. It may lead to the socially desirable change, in this case becoming more physically active, or not, or even to another prompt for deliberation.

These insights draw attention to the complexity and contingence of action, including actions designed to improve health and physiological function. The turn to PA and SB appears to represent a significant change in how we expect current and future lives to be led, what levels and quality of reflexivity we expect social actors to engage in. Indeed we might even suggest that the target of PA and SB recommendations is the internal conversation itself, and this level of intimate scrutiny must therefore be subjected to sociological analysis.

The problem of and with sitting

So far we have identified a range of insights and concepts, which provide us with the tools to critically analyse PA and SB. To continue this process of analysis, we can turn to some evidence. The focus therefore moves to how this new medical problem, named Sedentary Behaviour, is constructed in the recent literature on SB published in scientific and professional outlets. I undertook a search of articles available through Medline within the 2008–2014 time period. The search terms were 'sedentary lifestyles'[1] and 'age'. I obtained 2,000 results, from which I retained papers that dealt with adults and older adults. My focus was on how SB was operationalised, problematised and what solutions to the problem were proposed. Thus, the final number of articles retained for the analysis was 49.

The analysis was interpretive but also discursive: I sought to understand what descriptive techniques were used to assert the truth of SB as an urgent medical problem, which required the deployment of resources. Inevitably the analysis was also a search for what was left unsaid or skated over. Several themes emerged from the analysis: (1) the articulation of SB as a global problem, (2) the defining of SB as (part of) a lifestyle and its correlates, (3) the role of measurement in SB coming to existence and (4) the responsibility of experts in the fight against SB.

A global problem

I want to take a detour to a 2012 issue of the *Lancet* with a section dedicated to PA. It was meant as a global wake-up call. In this issue Das and Horton (2012: 189) posed the problem of what they called Physical Inactivity (PI) in the following terms: 'There is substantial evidence to show that PI is a major contributor to death and disability from non-communicable diseases (NCD) worldwide'. In the same issue, Wen and Wu (2012: 192) stated that 'inactive people are contributing to a mortality burden as large as tobacco smoking'.

The problem of PI is thus global. Its detrimental health effects are emphasised as are the consequences on health care systems. This position is reflected in the rest of the science literature. Indeed the scale of the problem is conveyed in the use of language which constructs it as a pandemic, making the need to address it urgent (Weiler, 2013), some authors even employing a war metaphor, encapsulated in Dibble and Billinger's (2013) title of their editorial article, 'On the Front Lines but not Engaged in the Battle', to coax health care professionals into action. The comparison of SB with smoking serves not only to reinforce the scale of the problem, but also perhaps its moral dimension. Suffice it to say that what we have here is the catastrophisation of inactivity. The emergence of the term 'sedentary behaviour' as the condition's official disease name is worthy of attention. Neville Owen, an Australian scientist, is a key figure in the transformation of PI into SB, having established its physiological correlates (see for instance Owen et al., 2010). Thus I now turn to the issues of naming and phenotyping.

SB as lifestyle

Being sedentary is a problem in its own right according to Brown (2013), characterised by being insufficiently active and from sitting too much. Sitting is a complex 'behaviour', with its own taxonomy, of which it is the genus and *prolonged* sitting is a specific manifestation of it. Prolonged sitting takes place in passive leisure, mostly TV viewing, as well as car, plane or train commuting and occupational sitting. There is a debate about the status of standing, which Owen et al. (2010) argue demands some metabolic expenditure, compared with sitting which deploys none. Thus, SB refers to a newly discovered phenotype, people who sit too much.

Excess sedentary sitting (Du et al., 2013) is habitual (Rutten et al., 2013), and Fioravanti (2012) and Bermúdez et al., (2013) refer to it as 'sedentarism'. Arguably the – ism suffix could simply be the way to turn the adjective sedentary into a noun. According to the Merriam-Webster dictionary (online), the suffix can fulfil three purposes: (1) To denote a practice or process, (2) To describe a condition or property and (3) To refer to a doctrine or belief system. All three definitions could potentially be applied. Indeed there is close conceptual proximity between sedentary-ism and lifestyle, which points to the key role attributed to individuals in the management of their health and the attainment of appropriate life regimes.

SB has health effects which are independent of PA behaviour (Owen et al., 2010). The correlates of PI act as its constitutive features and its consequences. Weight gain is the most frequently cited correlate of SB. High BMI, adiposity, hip to waist ratio and obesity are used interchangeably in all the papers reviewed as the visible manifestation of contemporary living worldwide (Du et al., 2013). Also, diet is often included. Carrère et al. (2013) cite unhealthy eating habits and insufficient PA as belonging to the same lifestyle as prolonged TV viewing. Burke et al. (2013) are searching for ways of encouraging behaviour change involving increases in PA and improved nutrition. SB is also associated, via weight gain, to cardio-vascular disease (Chomistek et al., 2013). However it is not clear what the direction of the relationship is. In most publications, the assumed relationship is that SB are lifestyle predictors of obesity or secondary ageing (for example Södergren, 2013). It is not the direction of association which is problematised, nor its existence, but how to get people to sit less – and thus to watch less TV. I now turn to the literature that deals with interventions and, relatedly, measurement.

Measurement and intervention

These two issues are interlinked. Measurement provides the empirical evidence that SB is real and also that interventions are effective. The next step is to embed the prescription of intervention into professional practice. Measurement, that is numbers, provides a baseline against which to determine abnormal, that is, pathological, sitting/inactivity. Measurement presents a set of problems however. Firstly, the scale must be capable of showing a measurable health outcome (SB=poor health, PA=good health), which has statistical significance. In other words, SB exists only insofar as it can be shown to have pathological consequences. Secondly, it must have reliability and validity. Thirdly, it must be usable as an aid to support epidemiological 'surveillance' (Clark et al., 2013). Fourthly, it must also help achieve behaviour change. Thus, measurement is at once a technical problem (how to) and a functional problem (what for). The question of how to measure SB is therefore central to its existence and its construction as a health-related lifestyle.

The responsibility of experts in the fight against SB

Colley et al. (2011) operationalise SB using accelerometers designed to provide data on time spent (that is, number of days and minutes) being sedentary and in a sliding scale of movement from light to vigorous and the number of steps taken per day. The use of technology is not universal: Clark et al. (2013) have tested women's past day recall of their sedentary time, that is their TV or screen time, as a valid and reliable measure of SB. However, technology is functional for intervention. For instance, Dobbins et al. (2013) propose developing digital technologies to help older people self-evaluate their SB. Bouchard et al. (2013) want to use technology to retrain older adults by recalibrating their own evaluation of PA intensity. In other words, it is hypothesised that older people's inactivity is the result of inappropriate or skewed knowledge about the sensory experience of their bodies in motion. Addressing SB means colonising people's lives in ways which mirror smoking or diet interventions: Rutten et al. (2013: 1) recommend prompts to get people to stand up every 30 minutes and thus swap a habit for another habitual response of 'getting up, and thus break up and reduce sitting time'.

Having identified the techniques which have brought SB into existence – as an urgent problem requiring professional intervention – I now turn to an examination of what this tells us about being old in contemporary society.

Bio-ethical agency

This critical review of recent PA and SB literature is instructive in several ways: it reflects the almost seismic shift in age-appropriate norms of living which has taken place in recent scientific work. The science, in its appropriation of sitting, has asserted its stronghold over our understanding of ageing and the provision of instructions on how to conduct our lives as we get old. This ensures the almost total capture of aged lives by science. The science of SB fills out the gaps left by PA recommendations. The molecular probing, which has enabled PA to become a legitimate prescription for secondary ageing, legitimises the extension of focus to SB.

Now the body has to be in perpetual motion, no longer a body of rest, but in restless, hyperactive mode. In other words, the everyday life of the aged body is colonised, known and monitored by measurement, given the proverbial kick up the backside using digital devices. The operationalisation of SB as prolonged sitting and TV or screen viewing is the moralisation of doing nothing, seated loitering without intent! Here we also see that the aged body is caught between two modalities of subjection: the imperative of healthy, thus ageless and timeless, ageing and the submission of everyday life to reflexive calculation.

As a behaviour, sitting not only leads to pathology, it becomes pathological in its own right. That is to say, its pathological status is confounded with its health consequences. The science of SB has power effects, which shape the reality of the body (Pronger, 2002). Older adults become caught up in a discursive grid with a tighter and more comprehensive reach, in which sitting and other behaviours can be correlated through the exclusive prism of health. In this space, acts of agency such as sitting, eating, watching TV, not fulfilling PA recommendations, are constructed as self-generated lifestyles in need of reform. The role of experts in the identification of the disease but also its treatment is central. To adapt Gilroy's insights (1989), power is EmBodied via physical activity and sedentary behaviour.

At least two important elements are elided in the reframing of sitting as behaviour and as part of a lifestyle. Firstly, lifestyles are outcomes of particular structural, cultural and individual circumstances. Using Archer's (2003) conceptualisation, we could say that the morphogenetic processes which cause aged lives to develop as they do are absent from the epistemology of SB. Secondly, the exclusive construction of sitting as negative and health-related behaviour bypasses the agential deliberations in which social actors engage in the privacy of their inner lives. These deliberations, informed by experience and undertaken in specific structural and cultural conditions may, or indeed may not, resolve 'the dilemma of [any] conflicting desires' (Archer, 2003: 27).

Rethinking PA and SB as an ethics of living

The ethnographic research on Masters sports demonstrates that physical dispositions in old age can be fundamentally reshaped. However, this outcome is the result of time-bound and contingent processes, the success or durability of which is never assured. The instability of PA can be extended to SB recommendations, as these require not only a fundamental reframing of everyday life, but also an instrumental, calculated and calculable, approach to the conduct of life. Thus, the construction of inactivity as behaviour and lifestyle creates a new subject position: the sedentary older person whose dispositional make-up must be transformed.

The creation of this new subject position does represent a 'vital politics', the implications of which must be examined in further research. Indeed, this process raises the following questions: how will people respond to the catastrophisation of their lives? What reflections on ageing and mortality will the recommendation to stand up for fitness (Rutten et al., 2013) elicit? The challenge now is to turn the medicalisation of PA and SB into an ethics which privileges people's own questioning, deliberations and solutions about their physicality, not necessarily to attain the correct body, but to negotiate an acceptable balance between one's conflicting wishes and desires.

Note

1. A search using the term sedentary* turned out not to be possible, which is perhaps of significance.

References

Archer MS (2003) *Structure, Agency and the Internal Conversation*. Cambridge: Cambridge University Press.
Bermúdez VJ, Rojas JJ, Córdova EB, Añez R, Toledo A, Aguirre MA, et al. (2013) International physical activity questionnaire overestimation is ameliorated by individual analysis of the scores. *American Journal of Therapeutics* 20(4): 448–458.
Bouchard DR, Langlois MF, Boisvert-Vigneault K, Farand P, Paulin M and Baillargeon JP (2013) Pilot study: can older inactive adults learn how to reach the required intensity of physical activity guideline? *Clinical Intervention in Aging* 8: 501–508.
Brown S (2013) Sitting is the problem, not just lack of exercise. *Menopause International* 19(2): 56–57.
Burke L, Lee AH, Jancey J, Xiang L, Kerr DA, Howat PA, et al. (2013) Physical activity and nutrition behavioural outcomes of a home-based intervention program for seniors: a randomized controlled trial. *The International Journal of Behavioral Nutrition and Physical Activity* 10: 14–14.
Carrère P, Atallah A, Kelly-Irving M, Lang T and Inamo J (2013) Television viewing and cardiovascular risk behaviors in the adult population of the French West Indies. *Annales de Cardiologie et d'Angeiologie* 62(3): 161–165.
Chomistek AK, Manson JE, Stefanick ML, Lu B, Sands-Lincoln M, Going SB, et al. (2013) Relationship of sedentary behavior and physical activity to incident cardiovascular disease: results from the Women's Health Initiative. *Journal of the American College of Cardiology* 61(23): 2346–2354.
Clark BK, Winkler E, Healy GN, Gardiner GN, Dunstan DW, Owen N, et al. (2013) Adults' past-day recall of sedentary time: reliability, validity, and responsiveness. *Medicine and Science in Sports and Exercise* 45(6): 1198–1207.
Colley RC, Garriguet D, Janssen I, Craig CL, Clarke J and Tremblay MS (2011) Physical activity of Canadian adults: accelerometer results from the 2007 to 2009 Canadian Health Measures Survey. *Health Reports* 22(1): 7–14.
Das P and Horton R (2012) Rethinking our approach to physical activity. *The Lancet* 380(9838): 189–190.
Dibble L and Billinger S (2013) On the front lines but not engaged in the battle. *Journal of Neurologic Physical Therapy: JNPT* 37(2): 49–50.
Dobbins C, Fergus P, Stratton G, Rosenberg M and Merabti M (2013) Monitoring and reducing sedentary behavior in the elderly with the aid of human digital memories. *Telemedicine Journal and E-Health: The Official Journal of the American Telemedicine Association* 19(3): 173–185.
Du H, Bennett D, Li L, Whitlock G, Guo Y, Collins R, et al. (2013) Physical activity and sedentary leisure time and their associations with BMI, waist circumference, and percentage body fat in 0.5 million adults: the China Kadoorie Biobank study. *The American Journal of Clinical Nutrition* 97(3): 487–496.

Estes CL (1979) *The Aging Enterprise: A Critical Examination of Social Policies and Services for the Aged*. San Francisco: Jossey Bass.
Fioravanti CH (2012) Brazilian fitness programme registers health benefits. *The Lancet* 380(9838): 206.
Foucault M (1997) The ethics of the concern for self as a practice of truth. In: Rabinow P (ed.) *Ethics: Subjectivity and Truth, the Essential Works*. London: Allen Lane.
Frankfurt HG (2004) *The Reasons of Love*. Princeton, NJ: Princeton University Press.
Fuller S (2011) *Humanity 2.0: What it Means to be Human Past, Present and Future*. Basingstoke: Palgrave.
Gilroy S (1989) The EmBody-ment of power: gender and physical activity. *Leisure Studies* 8: 163–171.
Hamilton MT, Healy GM, Dunstan DW, Zderic TW and Owen N (2008) Too little exercise and too much sitting: inactivity physiology and the need for new recommendations on sedentary behavior. *Current Cardiovascular Risk Reports* 2(4): 292–298.
Katz S (2013) Active and successful aging: lifestyle as a gerontological idea. *Recherches Sociologiques et Anthropologiques* 1: 53–75.
Merriam-Webster (online) http://www.merriam-webster.com/dictionary/ism (accessed February 2015).
Owen N, Healy GN, Matthews CE and Dunstan DW (2010) Too much sitting: the population-health science of sedentary behavior. *Exercise and Sport Sciences Review* 38(3): 105–116.
Peterson A and Bunton R (1997) *Foucault, Health and Medicine*. London: Routledge.
Pronger B (2002) *Body Fascism: Salvation in the Technology of Physical Fitness*. Toronto: University of Toronto Press.
Rose N (2007) *The Politics of Life itself: Biomedicine, Power, and Subjectivities in the 21st Century*. Princeton, NJ: Princeton University Press.
Rose N (1999) *Powers of Freedom*. Cambridge: Cambridge University Press.
Rutten GM, Savelberg HH, Biddle SJH and Kremers SPJ (2013) Interrupting long periods of sitting: good STUFF. *The International Journal of Behavioral Nutrition and Physical Activity* 10: 1–1.
Södergren M (2013) Lifestyle predictors of healthy ageing in men. *Maturitas* 75(2): 113–117.
Tulle E (2008a) Acting your age? Sports science and the ageing body. *Journal of Aging* 22(4): 340–347.
Tulle E (2008b) *Ageing, the Body and Social Change: Running in Later Life*. Basingstoke: Palgrave.
Weiler R (2013) Do all health care professionals have a responsibility to prescribe and promote regular physical activity: or let us carry on doing nothing. *Current Sports Medicine Reports* 12(4): 272–275.
Wen CP and Wu X (2012) Stressing harms of physical inactivity to promote exercise. *The Lancet* 380(9838): 192–193.

3
Physical Activity and Narratives of Successful Ageing

Elizabeth C.J. Pike

Introduction

There is considerable research evidence that indicates that the process of ageing and those who belong to the older population have long been defined as a threat to social values and interests (Critcher, 2003). From Ancient Greece when old age (*geras*) was mostly viewed as ugly, mean and tragic, through to the Byzantine Empire, later life was believed to be accompanied by economic vulnerability, physical frailty and social marginality. Medieval societies often took a more positive stance that old age was the end of life's journey toward wisdom and redemption (Gilleard, 2002, 2007a, b). In modern neoliberal societies, the large 'baby boom' generation born after the second World War is now reaching retirement with expectations of long life, and they are variously described through powerful (if misleading) metaphors such as a tsunami or an 'apocalypse of ageing' (Haber, 2004: 515).

This chapter will take as its focus examples of what is argued to constitute successful ageing set against this backdrop of the perceived 'apocalypse', and the interplay of dominant messages about ageing with engagement in, and experiences of, physical activity in later life. I will attempt to make sense of the role of physical activity in later life by providing stories of ageing drawing on what Barthes (1975: 237) described as a 'prodigious variety of genres'. In this case, the narratives come from texts including policy documents and public health messages about the benefits of physical activity and media reports in neoliberal societies which often appear to unquestioningly accept the need for older members of the population to take individual responsibility for engaging in 'active ageing' in order to 'age well', such that this has become a new framework for, and norm of, ageing. I will then explore some fictional representations of ageing which reinforce these messages before presenting some examples of the 'lived experiences' of being physically active in later life, drawing on a combination of participant observation, semi-structured interviews and stories written and told by older people. I wanted to hear their stories in their own words in order to gain an in-depth understanding of people whose voices have not been widely heard and whose experiences may inform future policy and practice in making more appropriate provisions for older people's physical activity.

My work is informed by Erving Goffman's belief that sociology is something that should be 'done' by observing, and interacting with, people's lives (see Birrell and Donnelly, 2004). In particular, a central tenet of Goffman's work is that age has to be understood as something that is performed and made meaningful via interactions, which are framed by social situations and interconnected with corporeality (see Laz, 2003; Phoenix and Sparkes, 2009). The social frame provided by policy and fictional sources, and lived corporeal experiences of ageing, is explored in what follows.

Narratives of ageing in policy Documents

The ageing population has been presented as a risk to society in policies, media reports and even academic symposia with researchers, practitioners and policy makers indicating the impending socio-economic threat caused by the growing numbers of frail and dependent older persons (Blaikie, 1999). Policy makers have since presented a counter-narrative of positive and healthy ageing which includes a need to be physically active. Governmental anti-ageing campaigns, medical and social care experts, thus aim to keep people healthy and independent of the need for socio-economic support (see Dionigi, 2006; Dionigi and O'Flynn, 2007). In neoliberal societies, this risk narrative and counter-discourse are used to emphasise individual responsibility: older people should provide for their own needs while simultaneously avoiding overburdening the economy or welfare services (Pike, 2011a). This includes an expectation to maintain youthfulness and active citizenship for as long as possible (Bytheway, 1995; Vincent, 2003). Katz (1996) has described social policy that targets older people in this way as a gerontological web: 'to be old merely requires that one ages. However, to be part of a population of elderly persons requires that one be absorbed into a specific discourse of differentiation' through distinctive policies (Katz, 1996: 51). Neilson (2006: 151) has argued that targeting older people in this way to maintain a youthful appearance and lifestyle also provides the basis for a 'blossoming consumer market'. Many members of the ageing population buy into the narratives from a complex network of health and beauty industries telling them how they should look and behave as they grow older. A significant part of these policies and social norms is an expectation to maintain levels of physical activity into later life (see Pike, 2011a). For example, the UK Department of Health guidelines state what older people (those aged over 65) '*should*' do, which includes being 'active daily', 'undertake physical activity to improve muscle strength on at least two days a week', 'minimise the amount of time spent being sedentary (sitting) for extended periods' (Department of Health, Physical Activity, Health Improvement and Protection, 2011: 39).

In an earlier study, I described how many older people experienced this policy-targeting, providing the example of one woman, aged 64, who explained:

I am definitely more aware now about the benefits of regular exercise. The publicity is all around, and I am inundated with junk mail, charity begging letters, etc. all telling me the benefits. Our local council run promotions and now government is giving healthy living more exposure. (in Pike, 2011b: 186)

It is interesting to consider whether these policy messages are a form of benign manipulation which encourage people into behaving in the desired way by suggesting that this is what the majority of people are doing or whether it means that growing older is experienced within a framework of age fundamentalism with youthfulness presented as a totalizing ideology from which there is little chance of escape (for further discussion of this, see Higgs et al., 2009; Katz, 1996).

Goffman (1963) distinguished between a person's public or *social identity*, how people are identified and categorised by others, and their private or *personal identity* constituted of those dimensions which make people distinctive from others. A key feature of the public aspects of ageing is that one's external appearance and behaviour is seen to say something about one's identity. In an interview, one 77-year-old woman described her lack of exercise as 'a failure of character' (in Pike, 2011b: 189), indicating that she felt an obligation to be more active because of the messages received from health campaigns and the media.

Interestingly, an unintended consequence of the emphasis on youthfulness in policy discourse and promotional materials appears to be an impression that 'You have to be young to do sport' (woman aged 74, in

Pike, 2011b: 192). This is a result of the dominant discourse of ageing as a period of frailty and decline combined with the youthful narratives presented in the health campaigns, which leads to contradictory messages as to whether the older person should avoid putting excessive pressures on their weakened bodies or should address their frailty influenced by the counter-discourse of positive/active/healthy ageing (see Phoenix and Grant, 2009). For some, this merely serves to encourage them to avoid physical activities that are inconsistent with their ageing habitus, or age-appropriate expectations (see Dionigi, 2006; Dionigi and O'Flynn, 2007; Dumas et al., 2005; Dumas and Turner, 2006). In the next section, I will discuss some of the fictional accounts of ageing that may influence what is seen as appropriate and possible with respect to engagement in physical activity in later life.

Fictional narratives of ageing

In a study of fictional narratives of ageing (Pike, 2013), I argue that fiction can be an important gerontological resource for understanding how ideas about ageing are shaped by culture, and how alternative images of ageing may be constructed and made possible through literary fiction (see Frank, 1995; Hepworth, 2000; Zeilig, 1997). This is in contrast to the more usual wariness of using fiction as a resource for academic study, as explained by Sandelowski (1991: 165): 'Anthropologist Clifford Geertz (1988: 140) noted the longstanding Western confusion of the imagined with the imaginary, the fictional with the false, and the making-things-out with making-things-up'.

Fictional representations of ageing were found to exaggerate and dramatise the negative narratives of ageing found in the policy documents described above. As Rebecca Solnit (2013: 150) writes in *The Faraway Nearby*, 'This is old age, the murderer of beauty, the ruin of vigor, the birthplace of sorrow, the grave of pleasure, the destroyer of memory'. Elsewhere, older people are portrayed as 'dependent, frail, vulnerable, poor, worthless, asexual, isolated, grumpy, behind the times, stupid, miserable, ga-ga, pathetic and a drain on society' (Healey and Ross, 2002: 110). With regards to fictional narratives of ageing and physical activity, most activities are portrayed as inappropriate or beyond the ability of the ageing body. For example, in fictional representations of physical activity in later life, we see that older people tend to be marginalised from the leisure activities of the younger people (see Pike, 2013). In Blake's (1789) *The Ecchoing Green,* the 'old folk' are literally on the sidelines watching the children at play:

Old John with white hair
Does laugh away care,
Sitting under the oak,
Among the old folk,
They laugh at our play,
And soon they all say.
Such such were the joys.
When we all girls & boys,
In our youth-time were seen,
On the Ecchoing Green.

However, I also found a more 'heroic' model of ageing than has been described previously: older people can engage in a variety of activities in later life if they so choose (see Reed et al., 2003). Perhaps the most well-known example of these is Father William's gymnastic leisure activities (Carroll, 1865: 45):

'"You are old, Father William," the young man said,
—"And your hair has become very white;
And yet you incessantly stand on your head –
—Do you think, at your age, it is right?"'

At this point, I turn my attention away from narratives of ageing presented in published documents to the lived experience of ageing as witnessed in participant observation and told to me during interviews and in written life stories. Interacting with older people's lives in this way enabled me to better understand how people view the ageing process, how this might be framed by published documents and how their subjective experiences influence lifestyle choices and may be used to inform social and health care practices.

The lived experience of 'defying old age'

In my work with members of Masters sports clubs, those referred to physical activity for health reasons and groups of older women, I have discovered inevitably varied experiences of the ageing process (Pike, 2011b, 2011c). The stories told to me ranged from those who were 'in tears' thinking about their failing body and impending mortality, to those who were 'defying old age' (see Pike, 2011b). Such stories are indicative of the progress that has been made in moving away from a blanket 'deficit model' of ageing (that ageing is only a negative experience and healthy ageing is simply the absence of disease) toward an alternative, positive 'heroic model' (that older people can, if they wish, engage in a whole range of activities into later life) (Reed et al., 2003; Tulle, 2008a, b, c).

It is evident that many older people are able to make pleasurable, active lifestyle choices in later life. This is particularly the case for those who benefit from the relative affluence of Western societies, whose social identities may be related to consumption (including of physical activities), as well as having access to health care. Blechman (2008) describes this as a form of 'Geritopia', or utopian way of growing old. For example, there are various older citizens' groups, television programmes such as 'Off Their Rockers' in which older people play pranks on the younger generation and 'Amazing Greys', which includes physical competitions between older and younger participants, 'The Zimmers' rock bank and the 'Company of Elders' dance group which are both constituted of older members, as well as Masters and Veterans sports competitions that offer considerable benefits to their participants. There are now a number of acronyms that have come into the vernacular to refer to the retired classes, including the WOOPIES: Well Off Older Persons; and the GLAMS: the Grey, Leisured And Moneyed.

In a study of Masters swimmers (Pike, 2011c), I describe the ways in which many used swimming as a means of impression management, to fend off the outer display, or 'mask of ageing' (Dionigi, 2002; Featherstone and Hepworth, 1991). In this way, they were able to defy an identity which was 'spoiled' by the ageing process in order to explore what they felt was their 'true' youthful self beneath the ageing exterior (Goffman, 1963, 1969). This is consistent with other research which argues that the engagement in 'cultures of fitness' is a way of resisting dominant ideologies and disassociating from the dependency and decline that is so often associated with ageing (see Paulson, 2005).

Some of the swimmers told stories of swimming in extreme environments which were 'all over the world' (male, age 70, in Pike, 2011c: 498), including 'every ocean I've visited from the tropics to the Arctic, remote rivers and lakes (male, age 64, in Pike, 2011c: 499). The adoption of lifestyles which are consistent with the sense of an inner youthful self, rather than the outer ageing self, have been described as strategies of masquerade (Biggs, 1993) or masquerades of youth (Woodward, 1991).

Some of the women in this study spoke quite specifically of the role of swimming in coping with the menopause. The menopause is a time in many women's lives when they feel and/or are considered 'old', unattractive in their decrepitude and of no use to society once they can no longer bear children (Vertinsky and O'Brien Cousins, 2007). The female Masters swimmers with whom I spoke described the positive role of swimming in negotiating this phase of their lives: 'I'm retired now, and hope to increase my exercising, as this really helps the side effects of the menopause and keeps my muscles flexible' (female, 60, in Pike, 2011c: 503).

In most cases, there was a 'use it or lose it' (male, aged 60) narrative expressed, indicating a fear of the alternatives – that to keep exercising is to avoid loss of health, independence, sense of self, even life (Dionigi, 2010). A caveat to these positive narratives is a concern expressed by Andrews (1999) that successful attempts to 'pass' as younger, may actually contribute to more subtle forms of ageism and the 'disappearance' of old age from public and social consciousness.

Being on 'the wrong side of an average'

In the final section of this paper, I present a short vignette, which connects the themes outlined in this chapter. In what follows, I set a lived experience of ageing against the backdrop of a fictional story and offer further comment on official discourse about the ageing process.

During the course of writing this chapter, I undertook a week's canoe expedition with three brothers, who in the year of the journey were aged 62, 60 and 55. I have written elsewhere about the appeal of outdoor adventurous activities as a means of facilitating successful ageing for some members of the older population (Pike and Weinstock, 2013). The experience reminded me of the tale of *Three Men in a Boat*. The men in this story were much younger but were still men who were 'feeling seedy' (Jerome, 1889: 5) and undertook the boat trip for the exercise and fresh air that they believed would improve their wellbeing. As with the fictional tale, we canoed down a river, camping along the route.

The river has often been used as a metaphor for life. Indeed, it could be argued that this is in itself an 'aged' metaphor, that like the river, life is a journey. Harrison (1995, cited in Fredin et al., 2004) argues that as with the life course, the river has a history, a source and an end, is always moving forward, starts small and gains substance along the route, is influenced by external forces and does not maintain a constant speed. In the poem *Ages of a River* (McBeath and Presswood, 2007), the river starts 'young and gurgling/thrown this way and that/by obstacles in the stream', 'moving rapidly/towards a destination' until it becomes 'slow, /meandering, /horizons ever broadening/we encounter you in the fullness/of older age'.

The brothers had canoed together from a very young age, and they reflected on their lives as they journeyed together down the river. At the beginning of the journey, the river was shallow, and the boat lurched as it hits rocks much like a young child learning to walk. Canoeing is physically demanding in these conditions, and during this period, there was considerable discussion of how 'you are just fitter when you are younger' (Morris, age 62) with the men making negative comparisons to their younger selves. Following Adler and Adler (1989), the ageing process is experienced as a loss of the former gloried athletic self. Each morning and evening, setting up camp and cooking food was interspersed with stretching exercises, complaints that 'everything aches' (Albert, age 60) and discussions of how their youthful squeals of excitement had been replaced by groans as they stood up, sat down and attempted to move around.

The middle part of the journey involved the negotiation of a series of rapids on the river. Harrison (1995) compares these to mid-life trials and tribulations, where it is necessary to react to surrounding forces. Conversations on these days turned to decisions about retirement (Morris was already retired; Albert and Willie were considering opportunities for early retirement). During one of these conversations, Albert reflected on official policies and discourse about the increasing numbers of older people in British society, such as those outlined earlier in this chapter, indicating that as he was less able to be physically active and required more from welfare services, so he felt that he was viewed by society as being on 'the wrong side of an average'.

The final day of the journey ended at the river mouth where the water flows more evenly than at its source in the mountains and dead trees that have been washed down the river lie in the river and on the banks as a stark reminder of the end of life. By this point in the journey, we had paddled for several days, wild camping on the river bank, and there were inevitable discussions about how old each of us felt. At the end of Jerome's (1889: 331) *Three Men in a Boat,* George is of the view that the trials and illnesses that had beset those three men suggested that they were journeying toward an inevitable death and had 'made up our minds to contract our certain deaths in this bally old coffin'. However, the sense of achievement on my journey with the three brothers also brought with it an optimism of a more heroic model of ageing as described above: 'being aged and achy just makes it better' (Willie, aged 55). Morris described how the ability to continue to be physically active had enabled him to 'grow old gracefully into my gardening years', and as they got out of the boats for the last time, he quoted Billy Connolly thanking his younger brothers for 'making a happy man very old'. The purpose of telling this story was to illustrate the challenges that are faced when attempting to maintain levels of physical activity into later life but also the positive experiences that this can bring. The messages from official sources, the media, and even fictional representations of ageing, tend to continue to be dominated by negative narratives and fear of what an ageing population means for society. However, the story of Morris, Albert and Willie tells us that even when you are engaging in physical activity while on 'the wrong side of an average', sometimes it 'just makes it better'.

References

Adler PA and Adler P (1989) The gloried self: the aggrandizement and the constriction of self. *Social Psychology Quarterly* 52(4): 299–310.
Andrews M (1999) The seductiveness of agelessness. *Ageing and Society* 19: 301–318.
Barthes R (1975) An introduction to the structural analysis of narrative. *New Literary History* 6(2): 237–272.
Biggs S (1993) *Understanding Ageing: Images, Attitudes and Professional Practice.* Buckingham, UK: Open University Press.
Birrell S and Donnelly P (2004) Reclaiming Goffman: Erving Goffman's influence on the sociology of sport. In: R Guilianotti (ed) *Sport and Modern Social Theorists.* Basingstoke: Palgrave MacMillan, pp.49–64.
Blaikie A (1999) *Ageing and Popular Culture.* Cambridge: Cambridge University Press.
Blake W (1789) *Songs of Innocence and Experience: Shewing the Two Contrary States of the Human Soul, 1789–1794.* Oxford: Oxford Paperbacks.
Blechman A (2008) *Leisureville: Adventures in America's Retirement Utopias.* New York: Atlantic Monthly Press.
Bytheway B (1995) *Ageism.* Buckingham, UK: Open University Press.
Carroll L (1865) *Alice's Adventures in Wonderland.* London: The Thames Publishing Co.
Critcher C (2003) *Moral Panics and the Media.* Buckingham, UK: Open University Press.
Department of Health, Physical Activity, Health Improvement and Protection (2011) *Start Active, Stay Active: A Report on Physical Activity from the Four Home Countries' Chief Medical Officers.* London: Department of Health, Physical Activity, Health Improvement and Protection.
Dionigi R (2010) Masters sport as a strategy for managing the ageing process. In: J Baker, S Horton and P Weir (eds) *The Masters Athlete: Understanding the Role of Sport and Exercise in Optimizing Aging.* London: Routledge, pp.137–156.
Dionigi R and O'Flynn G (2007) Performance discourses and old age: what does it mean to be an older athlete? *Sociology of Sport Journal* 24: 359–377.

Dionigi R (2006) Competitive sport and aging: the need for qualitative sociological research. *Journal of Aging and Physical Activity* 14: 365–379.
Dionigi R (2002) Leisure and identity management in later life: understanding competitive sport participation among older adults. *World Leisure Journal* 44: 4–15.
Dumas A and Turner B (2006) Age and ageing: the social world of Foucault and Bourdieu. In: J Powell and A Wahidin (eds) *Foucault and Ageing*. New York: Nova Publishers, pp.145–155.
Dumas A, Laberge S and Straka S (2005) Older women's relations to bodily appearance: the embodiment of social and biological conditions of existence. *Ageing and Society* 25: 883–902.
Featherstone M and Hepworth M (1991) The mask of ageing and the postmodern life course. In: M Featherstone, M Hepworth and B Turner (eds) *The Body*. London: Sage, pp.371–390.
Frank A (1995) *The Wounded Storyteller: Body, Illness, and Ethics*. Chicago: University of Chicago Press.
Fredin T, Hastie K and Champion B (2004) *Waters to the Sea*. Hamline University, US: The Center for Global Environmental Education.
Gilleard C (2007a) Old age in Ancient Greece: narratives of desire, narratives of disgust. *Journal of Aging Studies* 21(1): 81–92.
Gilleard C (2007b) Old age in Byzantine society. *Ageing and Society* 27(5): 623–642.
Gilleard C (2002) Aging and old age in Medieval society and the transition of modernity. *Journal of Ageing and Identity* 7(1): 25–41.
Goffman E (1969) *Where the Action Is*. London: The Penguin Press.
Goffman E (1963) *Stigma: Notes on the Management of Spoiled Identity*. Harmondsworth, UK: Penguin.
Haber C (2004) Life extension and history: the continual search for the fountain of youth. *Journal of Gerontology: Biological Sciences* 59(6): 515–522.
Healey T and Ross K (2002) Growing old invisibly: older viewers talk television. *Media, Culture and Society* 24: 105–120.
Hepworth M (2000) *Stories of Ageing*. Buckingham, UK: Open University Press.
Higgs P, Leontowitsch M, Stevenson F and Rees Jones I (2009) Not just old and sick: the 'will to health' in later life. *Ageing and Society* 29(5): 687–707.
Jerome J (1889) *Three Men in a Boat (To Say Nothing of the Dog)*. Bristol: JW Arrowsmith.
Katz S (1996) *Disciplining Old Age: The Formation of Gerontological Knowledge*. Charlottesville, VA: University of Virginia Press.
Laz C (2003) Age embodied. *Journal of Aging Studies* 17: 503–519.
McBeath C and Presswood T (2007) Ages of a river. Available at www.dancingscarecrow.org.uk.
Neilson B (2006) Anti-ageing cultures, biopolitics and globalisation. *Cultural Studies Review* 12(2): 149–164.
Paulson P (2005) How various 'cultures of fitness' shape subjective experiences of growing older. *Ageing and Society* 25: 229–244.
Phoenix C and Grant B (2009) Expanding the agenda for research on the physically active ageing body. *Journal of Aging and Physical Activity* 17: 362–379.
Phoenix C and Sparkes A (2009) Being Fred: big stories, small stories and the accomplishment of a positive ageing identity. *Qualitative Research* 9: 219–236.

Pike E (2013) The role of fiction in (mis)representing later life leisure activities. *Leisure Studies* 32(1): 69–88.

Pike E and Weinstock J (2013) Identity politics in the outdoor adventure environment. In: E Pike and S Beames (eds) *Social Theory and Outdoor Adventure*. London: Routledge, pp.125–134.

Pike E (2011a) The active ageing agenda, old folk devils and a new moral panic. *Sociology of Sport Journal* 28: 209–225

Pike E (2011b) Growing old (dis)gracefully? the gender/ageing/exercise nexus. In: E Kennedy and P Markula (eds) *Women and Exercise: The Body, Health and Consumerism*. London: Routledge, pp.180–196.

Pike E (2011c) Aquatic antiques: swimming off this mortal coil? *International Review for the Sociology of Sport* 47: 492–510.

Reed J, Cook G, Childs S and Hall A (2003) *Getting old is not for cowards: Comfortable, healthy ageing*. York: Joseph Rowntree Foundation.

Sandelowski M (1991) Telling stories: narrative approaches in qualitative research. *Journal of Nursing Scholarship* 23(2): 161–166.

Solnit R (2013) *The Faraway Nearby*. London: Granta.

Tulle E (2008a) Acting your age? sports science and the ageing body. *Journal of Aging Studies* 22(4): 340–347.

Tulle E (2008b) The ageing body and the ontology of ageing: athletic competence in later life. *Body and Society* 14: 1–19.

Tulle E (2008c) *Ageing, the Body and Social Change*. Basingstoke: Palgrave MacMillan.

Vertinsky P and O'Brien Cousins S (2007) Acting your age: gender, age and physical activity. In: P White and K Young (eds) *Gender and Sport in Canada*. Oxford: Oxford University Press, pp.155–193.

Vincent J (2003) *Old Age*. London: Routledge.

Woodward K (1991) *Aging and its Discontents: Freud and other Fictions*. Bloomington, IN: Indiana University Press.

Zeilig H (1997) The uses of literature in the study of older people. In: A Jamieson, S Harper and C Victor (eds) *Critical Approaches to Ageing and Later Life*. Buckingham, UK: Open University Press, pp.39–48.

4
Fitness and Consumerism in Later Life
Paul Higgs and Chris Gilleard

Introduction

While physical exercise has conventionally been associated with masculinity and youth, changes over the last half century have seen exercise become commoditised and incorporated into the ungendered discourses of 'active ageing' (Walker, 2008). Although physical exercise has long been part of the care and cultivation of the self (Foucault, 1986), its practices and meanings have changed over time. In contemporary society, exercise has become a more 'individualised', 'fashioned' aspect of lifestyle, a set of embodied practices through which social distinction is created and interpreted beyond the barriers of age and gender. Unlike the individualistic and gendered practices associated with cosmetics, fashion and hairstyle, however, physical exercise embodies public virtue as well as the agentic nature of social citizenship (Lupton, 1995). Its role as a public good has become central to public health campaigns promoting the message that health and fitness are civic virtues to be cultivated at all ages and among all groups, a necessary part of the war against 'indolence' represented by the 'obesity epidemic' and the diseases of affluence (Campos, 2004). This combination of consumerism and the individualisation of citizenship have contributed to the transformation of exercise and fitness beyond the boundaries of age.

Exercise and fitness

Though the link between virtue and fitness has a long history, the extension of the virtuous pursuit of exercise to later life is of recent origin. Much of the early physiological research on ageing and exercise was about assessing older men's fitness for work rather than their capacity to live longer or live better (Åstrand et al., 1959; Botwinick and Shock, 1952; Dawson and Hellebrandt, 1945). While the 'commercialisation' of exercise and fitness was present at the beginning of the twentieth century alongside their role in equipping the state with a disciplined military and productive workforce, women and the old were advised against any but the gentlest forms of exercise. Throughout the late nineteenth and early twentieth century, medical literature was used to constrain young women's participation in certain sports education and the majority of sports (Vertinsky, 1987) as well as to prevent older women's enjoyment of exercise. Exercise was thought to risk 'damaging' women's reproductive capacity, while in later life 'aging women were perceived to be invalids in need of care, lacking the necessary vital energy to participate in onerous daily activities' (Vertinsky, 1991: 77). Similar negative views about men's exercise in mid and later life were expressed well into the twentieth century as men over forty were advised – and seemed to accept – that they should avoid any vigorous exercise that risked assaulting their creaking joints and 'beat up' circulatory systems (Luciano, 2001: 58).

Things changed during the course of the second half of the twentieth century with the emergence of what Turner (1984) has called the 'somatic society'. Van Hilvoorde has described this period as producing 'a culture in which people motivated by a mix of cosmetic and medical concerns voluntarily and deliberately engage in physical exercises' (2008: 1320). The rise of a dual concern with appearance and health and well-being enabled a less gendered culture of fitness to emerge, standing in sharp contrast to the previous collectivised routines that had centred on youth, war and work fitness. Now these regimes were reconstituted as individualised activities aimed at making bodies whole, healthy and attractive. All of this was increasingly appealing to a growing global market in leisure goods and services. Fitness was becoming 'postmodern'. Indeed, Glassner has argued that fitness is quintessentially a postmodern condition where the appeal of fitness products and practices offer 'the opportunity to disenthrall [one's] self from the perceived shortcomings of everyday life in modern culture – in particular from constraining dualities such as expert versus amateur, self versus body, male versus female and work versus leisure (1989: 182). As a result, exercise has emerged as a desirable goal not just for youth, but for middle aged people too (Benson, 1997: 128). The 'middle-ageing' of the 'baby boomer' cohorts and their concern to stay young proved an important stimulus in this transformation, typified by the rise of aerobics, jogging and the work-out (Gilleard and Higgs, 2013: 135).

The discourses of fitness soon extended further and entered into later life. As Kagan and Morse (1988) have pointed out, previous socially orientated productivist and gendered concerns about fitness were 'displaced to a struggle within the body itself' where the implicit enemy was 'the body itself as it ages' (169). While the incorporation of a cosmetic and medical aesthetic into the new exercise regimes may have created new and gendered conflicts about outcomes it soon became clear that many men also shared these aspirations – especially in relation to the moral imperative to protect oneself from the ills of a society of excess by re-theorising notions of self-hood (Glassner, 1989).

The shift from collective to individualised approaches to fitness has also been seen as facilitating the commodification of exercise where exercise and fitness are seen as desirable individual goals promoting the social virtue of individualised health and fitness. Not only has exercise become an important dimension of social distinction in a somatic society, it is one that now operates as a civic imperative at all ages. Health promotion for what Deborah Lupton (1995) has termed the 'regulated body' repeatedly suggests that individual health is not only a personal concern, it is more or less a civic duty which operates through a 'will to health' that must be demonstrated at all points and in nearly all conditions. While this development has been closely identified with the rise of neo-liberal modes of health policy, it is also connected to the rise of citizenship as a form of governmentality (Higgs et al., 2009). For older people, their engagement with various 'technologies of the self' that are designed to promote fitness at later ages is set against the background of changing expectations of the norms that they are expected to reach with regard to their health and fitness. In part this is an extension of the 'polysemous' nature of the idea of fitness in a consumer society that we will explore in relation to the work of Zygmunt Bauman, but it is also a product of the collapse of the inter-relationship between normal ageing and the normativity of ageing. Older people increasingly exist in an environment where diversity is expected but which still creates normative expectations of what individuals are expected to do (Beck, 2007). Consequently, to use Mitchell Dean's distinction of the 'civilised' and the 'marginalised' (2007), we can see how a failure to engage with exercise and fitness can result in some individuals finding themselves transferred to a status of marginalisation.

Bauman, consumerism and fitness

The idea of fitness as a phenomenon of post-modernity espoused by Glassner (1989) is also explored in the work of Zygmunt Bauman. Going beyond a simple notion of fitness as an aspect of health, Bauman sees fitness as a defining feature of the somaticised consumer culture where the anxieties of a more contingent 'liquid modernity' are acted upon and recreated (2000). For Bauman the pursuit of fitness is much more than a peripheral aspect of people's lives, rather it acts as the organising principle for a whole range of social actions. He situates his argument by pointing out that modern society has moved from being a 'society of producers' to one that can be described as a 'society of consumers'. For him this is not just an economic transformation, it is also a thoroughgoing ontological transformation where each person's body becomes seen as the focus of individual action rather than being seen simply as a factor of production, reproduction or military might. He writes:

> The postmodern body is first and foremost a receiver of sensations, it imbibes and digests experiences; the capacity of being stimulated renders it an instrument of pleasure. That capacity is called fitness; obversely the 'state of unfitness' stands for languor, apathy, listlessness, dejection, a lackadaisical response to stimuli; for a shrinking or just 'below average' capacity for, and an interest in, new sensations and experiences. (1995:116)

The 'fitness' of the postmodern body, then, is central to the practices of contemporary consumerism setting up both discourses of 'engagement' and feelings of unease and dissatisfaction with that engagement. This has considerable benefits for a consumer culture where these feelings of dissatisfaction lead to a constant need to attempt to reach higher ideals of fitness irrespective of whatever level has been previously reached. In a significant passage Bauman writes:

> 'Fitness' is to a consumer in the society of consumers what 'health' was to the society of producers. It is a certificate of 'being in', of belonging, of inclusion, of the right of residence. 'Fitness' knows no upper limit; it is, in fact, defined by the absence of limit... However fit your body is – you could make it fitter. However fit it may be at the moment, there is always a vexing helping of 'unfitness' mixed in, coming to light or guessed at whenever you compare what you have experienced with the pleasures suggested by the rumors and sights of other people's joys which you have failed to experience thus far and can only imagine and dream of living through yourself. In the search for fitness, unlike in the case of health, there is no point at which you can say: now that I have reached it I may as well stop and hold onto and enjoy what I have. There is no 'norm' of fitness you can aim at and eventually attain. (2005: 93)

This view echoes Featherstone's (1991) idea of the 'performing self' who is driven by consumption and by the moral imperative to 'not to let one's self go' in an endless quest to enhance an individual's own health and marketability. Jones and Higgs (2010) have argued that this focus meshes with the culture of the third age through the effect of continually increased expectations being placed upon individuals in order that they can demonstrate both their 'will to health' and their capacity to engage with all manner of anti-ageing techniques in order to slow the evidence and problems associated with old age. Health and social policies are no longer the main influence on health in later life and have become one aspect of the older individual's engagement with the consumer market. Ideas of 'healthy' or 'successful' ageing can also be viewed in this prism which is reconstructed as a task for the reflexive 'older' self to act agentically by making the right choices for their future wellbeing in order to age without disease, dysfunction or indeed, any diminishment of self (Higgs, 2012). As Jones and Higgs (2010) point out, the drive to demonstrate fitness at older ages becomes a new normativity separating out those capable of maintaining a position in the third age from those becoming increasingly defined by the discourses of the fourth age. Instead of an overarching 'natural' ageing accommodating all those deemed to be old, a fragmenting of the various statuses and stages of later life is encouraged by state and market alike. This is done in part to ensure that 'consumers' can be separated from 'proxy consumers' in order to maximise both market penetration for those able to demonstrate a state of agentic 'agelessness' and market optimisation for those deemed to have lost that capacity.

Because of the role that a concentration on exercise and health in later life seems to have on the moral value of old age, some gerontologists have adopted what they term an 'anti-anti-ageing' position as a way of critiquing the commoditisation of anti-ageing approaches (Vincent et al., 2008). Unlike past views about the unsuitability of exercise in later life, the new critique of exercise as 'anti-ageing' is often ambivalent about it. This view may reflect a general wish to both promote an ideal of 'healthy ageing' as an individual and public virtue while descrying the promotion of a 'fit' body in later life as a signifier of fashion driven consumerism. The anti-ageing properties of exercise are criticised for creating the narrative fiction of 'a new older adult, strong, trainable with improved psychological and health status' (Tulle, 2008: 344) which thus imagined, brings into contrast, oppresses even, those who, ageing unsuccessfully, demonstrate their abjection before the motif of the 'master athlete'. This conflict between acceptance of ageing and old age and those who have expanding possibilities of not appearing or not performing as old becomes a key line of fracture in understanding old age. Calasanti and Slevin (2001) posit this as a moral issue: Individuals not only can, but should exert control over their ageing. However, as we have seen, others see this differently. The narratives of the master athlete embody a desired extension of life not dominated by oldness and agedness, one which replaces decline with increased physical performance and the pursuit of competitive advantage displayed in the contemporary institutionalisation of 'the master athlete'.

Ageing, fitness and the exercise of virtue

Ageless physical activity is more than a deliberate tactic of seeking distinction and power through 'age resistance'. It is part of a broader social response to the changing balance between work and leisure, reflecting what Bauman has characterised as a shift from a society of producers to a society of consumers. As work as the exertion of physical labour has declined in the most prosperous nations, compensatory routines have come into play in the form of 'active' leisure which has increasingly become part of consumer society. Unlike work-dependent patterns of physical activity, active leisure can be more easily extended beyond the circumstances of working life. When the end of work meant the end of labour, more often than not it meant an inactive retirement – hence retirement being framed as a tragedy or loss. But by the late 1970s and early 1980s, the inactivity of retirement was replaced by the new 'busy ethic' of leisure (Ekerdt et al., 1988). Formerly proscribed, exercise and activity in mid-life and in retirement began to be positively promoted. In 1972, less than half the Finnish population in their fifties were physically active in their leisure time; by 1992, that figure had risen to just over three quarters (Borodulin et al., 2008). No longer forced to labour, older bodies were now exercised with care, but within the context of active leisure. For those no longer working, later life has become progressively more active, with recent retirees exercising more than retirees from earlier cohorts (Agahi and Parker, 2005; Cozijnsen et al., 2014; Petersen et al., 2010).

The full extent of this change can be seen in European comparisons of sporting activity conducted a half century or so apart. In a 1953 Danish national survey of over 1000 adults, less than 10% of those aged over 50 reported any active engagement with sport, with most reporting none or only a passive engagement as spectators (Andersen et al., 1956). In 2003, the German National Health Interview found that some 30% of men and 22% of women *in their seventies* reported participating in at least two hours of sporting activities per week, the most popular activities being cycling, gymnastics and swimming (Hinrichs et al., 2010). Numerous national surveys and reports of health and physical activity still indicate a gendered imbalance in the number of men and women engaging in sports and other deliberate physical activities, at all stages of life. But increasingly this is a difference in the pattern rather than the overall level of participation. Thus 'individualised' regimes of exercise such as walking, swimming, jogging and cycling are practiced more often by older men while aerobic, gymnastic and related group fitness activities are practiced more often by older women (Tischer et al., 2011), although there is evidence that all gender differences are declining (Borodulin et al., 2008).

The investment in the body pursued through these various exercise and sports regimes is realised in and through the market. This may include going to commercial organisations such as private gyms, leisure centres, aerobic dance classes or various not-for-profit social clubs or using commercial products such as workout regimes on videos or DVDs, computer exercise games, smart phone 'activity and fitness' applications, cycling, rowing or similar fitness machines, treadmills and other forms of exercising machinery. Some form of 'home trainer' for example can be found in over 30% of later life German households (Gilleard and Higgs, 2011: 365). While pensioners clubs and other local government settings may still offer free fitness classes, such settings can be seen as the failed choices of the marginalised rather than the preferred later life styles of successful consumers.

Fitness is consequently more than the exercise of a consumerist interpellation. If one pursues the idea that ageing is at bottom no more than the consequence of an inadequate genetic investment in the soma, as Kirkwood among others have implied (Kirkwood, 1997), compensating for this lack of genetic investment by investing in a refashioned lifestyle seems a logical response. Within the paradigm of what Gilleard and Higgs (2013) have called 'the new ageing', exercise and fitness oriented practices can be seen as deliberate social and cultural investment in embodied practices oriented toward 'not becoming old'. The success of which is both a source of distinction and individualised moral virtue.

Conclusions

The pursuit of fitness in later life has become part of the new ageing ethic embodied in the ideals of active, productive or successful ageing.

In this chapter, we have used the term 'exercise' to cover what are in fact a wide variety of embodied practices ranging from body building to walking, marathon running to step and dance aerobics. What distinguishes the physical exercise regimes of first modernity from those of second modernity is the latter's individualisation, commercialisation and integration into the broader 'lifestyles' of those no longer young. In other words, becoming part of consumer society. Jogging and aerobics, home trainers and DVD fitness exercises, computerised 'activity' games and the complex electronic devices used to monitor progress target the individual consumer of all ages are all part of the evidence of the role of consumption in constructing fitness. The expanding keep fit industry vastly overshadows that of the old-fashioned body building regimes of Eugen Sandow in the 1900s and the 'dynamic tension' methods promoted by Charles Atlas in the dying decades of first modernity.

The individualisation of fitness has also promoted, or at least facilitated, less exclusionary practices with respect both to gender and age. Aerobics, jogging, marathons and work-outs are as accessible to those in mid and later life as they are to those still young and, increasingly, as much to women as to men (Tischer et al, 2011). This is true not just for the more 'cosmetic' forms of fitness involved in work-outs and aerobics, but for those activities where master athletes compete. Over the last three decades, for example, older women have increased their participation in the New York City marathon, more than any other demographic group (Lepers and Cattagni, 2012).

As exercise oriented body-work has moved from the realms of production to those of leisure and consumption, it has more easily been incorporated into leisured later lifestyles. While the forms of physical activity undertaken by older bodies are still connected with the embodied identities of gender, race and disability, they are less connected to the productive processes of society. Their old embodied identities do not so much constrain as segment the market. This is not to ignore that as participation in exercise and fitness becomes an expanding new virtuous 'norm', issues of distinction become issues of marginalisation, as failure to demonstrate an engagement with health promoting forms of exercise becomes a marker of a personal failure to become self-constituting and agentic (Jones and Higgs 2010). Following Lupton's 'imperative of health' (1995), whatever the personal outcome, it is necessary to acknowledge the reality of the cultural shift towards the need to 'exercise' the body in later life irrespective of the consequences that follow.

It is also important to recognise that there is no single discourse associated with exercise, just as there is no single consumerist voice. The practice of fitness is polysemous. It is shaped by history as much as by gender or chronological age. It reinforces some aspects of identity as well as undermining or denying others. Exercise can be seen as part of the anti-ageing enterprise, an alternative cosmetics of the body, colluding with and reinforcing a fear of ageing that permeates the cultures of second modernity (Vincent et al., 2008: 293). At the same time, it can be seen as part of modern bio politics whereby the internalisation of bodily standards and regimes enables responsibility for one's own 'bodily good condition' to be shifted from the state and society to the individual and his or her household (Higgs et al, 2010). But, as Phoenix and Smith (2011) have pointed out, the 'counter-stories' of master athletes can also contribute to 'new aging identities' that can 'evoke social change in the way that aging is interpreted and given meaning' (637). Viewed in this light, exercise represents a form of performativity resisting the performer's objectification as 'aged' and his or her oppression by the community of 'old age' (Sims-Gould et al., 2010). Adopting one of Foucault's later formulations, exercise and physical activity can be seen as part of the agonistic exploration both of what human bodies can be, and what they can become (Foucault, 1982). And of course exercise can also be a way of people having fun, enjoying being a body that both performs and serves a positive sense of self without reference to age (Tulle, 2008).

References

Agahi N and Parker MG (2005) Are today's older people more active than their predecessors? Participation in leisure-time activities in Sweden in 1992 and 2002. *Ageing and Society* 25(6): 925–941.
Andersen H, Bo-Jensen A, Elkær-Hansen N and Sonne A (1956) Sports and games in Denmark in the light of sociology. *Acta Sociologica* 2(1): 1–27.
Åstrand I, Åstrand PO and Rodahl K (1959) Maximal heart rate during work in older men. *Journal of Applied Physiology* 14: 562–566.
Bauman Z (1995) *Life in Fragments*. London: Basil Blackwell.
Bauman Z (2000) *Liquid Modernity*. Cambridge: Polity.
Bauman Z (2005) *Liquid Life*. Cambridge: Polity.
Beck U (2007) Beyond class and nation: reframing social inequalities in a globalizing world. *The British Journal of Sociology* 58(4): 679–705.
Benson J (1997) *Prime Time: A History of the Middle Aged in Twentieth-Century Britain*. London: Longman.
Borodulin K, Laatikainen T, Juolevi A and Jousilahti P (2008) Thirty-year trends of physical activity in relation to age, calendar time and birth cohort in Finnish adults. *European Journal of Public Health* 18(3): 339–344.
Botwinick J and Shock, NW (1952) Age differences in performance decrement with continuous work. *Journals of Gerontology* 7(1): 41–46.

Calasanti TM and Slevin KF (2001) *Gender, Social Inequalities and Aging*. Walnut Creek, California: AltaMira Press.
Campos PF (2004). *The obesity myth: Why America's obsession with weight is hazardous to your health*. New York: Penguin.
Cooper KH (1970) *New Aerobics*. New York: Bantam Press.
Cozijnsen R, Stevens NL, and Van Tilburg TG (2013) The trend in sport participation among Dutch retirees, 1983–2007. *Ageing and Society* 33(04): 698–719.
Dawson PM and Hellebrandt FA (1945) The influence of aging in man upon his capacity for physical Work and upon his cardio-vascular response to exercise. *American Journal of Physiology* 143(3): 420–427.
Dean M (2007) *Governing Societies*. Buckingham, UK: Open University Press.
Dinnerstein M and Weitz R (1994) Jane Fonda, Barbara Bush and other aging bodies: femininity and the limits of resistance. *Feminist Issues* 14(2): 3–24.
Foucault M (1982) The subject and power. In: HL Dreyfuss and P Rabinow (eds) *Michel Foucault: Beyond Structuralism and Hermeneutics*. Hemel Hempstead, UK: Harvester Wheatsheaf, pp. 208–226.
Foucault M (1986) *The History of Sexuality, Volume Three: The Care of the Self* R Hurley (trans). London: Penguin Books.
Gilleard C and Higgs P (2011) Consumption and aging. In: R Setterson and JL Angel (eds) *Handbook of Sociology of Aging*. New York: Springer, pp.361–375.
Gilleard C and Higgs P (2013) *Ageing, Corporeality and Embodiment*. London: Anthem Press.
Glassner B (1989) Fitness and the postmodern self. *Journal of Health and Social Behavior* 30(6): 180–191.
Higgs P (2012) Consuming bodies: Zygmunt Bauman on the difference between fitness and health. In G Scambler (ed) *Contemporary Theorists for Medical Sociology*. London: Routledge, pp. 20–32.
Higgs P, Leontowitsch M, Stevenson F and Jones IR (2009) Not just old and sick: the will to health in later life. *Ageing and Society* 29:687–707.
Hinrichs T, Trampisch U, Burghaus I, Endres HG, Klaaßen-Mielke R, Moschny A, et al. (2010) Correlates of sport participation among community-dwelling elderly people in Germany: a cross-sectional study. *European Review of Aging and Physical Activity* 7: 105–115.
Jones IR and Higgs P (2010) The natural, the normal and the normative: contested terrains in ageing and old age. *Social Science and Medicine* 71(8): 1513–1519.
Kagan E and Morse M (1988) The body electronic: aerobic exercise on video: women's search for empowerment and self-transformation. *TDR* 32(4): 164–180.
Kirkwood T (1997) The origins of human ageing. *Philosophical Transactions of the Royal Society of London Series B-Biological Sciences* 352(1363): 1765–1772
Lepers R and Cattagni T (2012) Do older athletes reach limits in their performance during Marathon running? *Age* 34(3):773–81.
Luciano L (2001) *Looking Good: Male Body Image in Modern America*. New York: Hill and Wang.
Lupton D (1995) *The Imperative of Health: Public Health and the Regulated Body*. London: Sage.
Petersen CB, Thygesen LC, Helge JW, Grønbæk M and Tolstrup JS (2010) Time trends in physical activity in leisure time in the Danish population from 1987 to 2005. *Scandinavian Journal of Public Health* 38(2): 121–128.

Phoenix C and Smith B (2011) Telling a (good?) counter story of aging: natural bodybuilding meets the narrative of decline. *The Journals of Gerontology, Series B: Psychological and Social Sciences* 66(5): 628–639.

Sims-Gould J, Clarke LH, Ashe MC, Naslund J and Liu-Ambrose T (2010) Renewal, strength and commitment to self and others: older women reflections of the benefits of exercise using Photovoice. *Qualitative Research in Sports and Exercise* 2(2): 250–266.

Tischer U, Hartmann-Tews I and Combrink C (2011) Sport participation of the elderly: the role of gender, age and social class. *European Review of Aging and Physical Activity* 8(1): 83–91.

Tulle E (2008) Acting your age? sports science and the ageing body. *Journal of Aging Studies* 22(4): 340–347.

Turner BS (1984) *The Body and Society*. Oxford: Basil Blackwell.

Van Hilvoorde I (2008) Fitness: the early (Dutch) roots of a modern industry. *The International Journal of the History of Sport* 25(10): 1306–1325.

Vertinsky P (1987) Exercise, physical capability and the eternally wounded woman in late nineteenth century North America. *Journal of Sport History* 14(1): 7–27.

Vertinsky P (1991) Old age, gender and physical activity: The biomedicalization of aging. *Journal of Sport History* 18(1): 64–80.

Vincent J, Tulle E and Bond J (2008) The anti-aging enterprise: science, knowledge, expertise, rhetoric and values. *Journal of Aging Studies* 22(4): 291–294.

Walker A (2008) Commentary: the emergence and application of active aging in Europe. *Journal of Aging and Social Policy* 21(1): 75–93.

5
Type 2 Diabetes and Commitment of Seniors to Adapted Physical Activity within the French System of Therapeutic Education

Nathalie Barth and Claire Perrin

Introduction

While the ageing of the population can in part be attributed to improvements in the field of health, it also raises new issues. Contemporary ageing tends to be characterised by greater sedentariness, exacerbated by loneliness and the loss of social contact. This often results in a decrease in function (decreased muscle strength, responsiveness, reflex and precise gestures, breathing capacity), which in turn increases the risk of developing chronic pathologies (cardiovascular illnesses, type 2 diabetes, hypertension, osteoarthritis, and so forth), compounding ageing processes. The aim is not only to add years to a person's life, but also to add life to those years by sustaining autonomy for as long as is possible. This is considered to be the key to successful ageing and physical activity the key to autonomy (Henaff-Pineau, 2009: 82). The scientifically established therapeutic and prevention benefits of regular physical exercise for ageing and chronic pathologies underpin the development of exercise adapted in accordance with the objectives (Perrin, 2008, 2012; Sparkes et al., 2012; Tulle, 2012, Poortmans and Carpentier, 2009). The various 'Ageing Well' programmes (*Programme Nationaux Nutrition Santé* [PNNS 1 and 2, Ministère de la santé et des solidarités] and *Bien Vieillir* 2003–2007 and 2007–2009 [Ministère de la santé et des solidarités]) promoting active ageing are nevertheless difficult to implement among a sedentary senior population suffering from an array of chronic pathologies. Associated with reduced physical capabilities, ageing alone is, in fact, likely to constitute an obstacle to regular physical exercise (Tulle, 2012; Feillet, 2000; Nicolson, 2004). Old people 'tend[ed] to continue their activities regardless of changes in work and age', with the exception of 'those who stopped working because of an illness experience' (Scherger et al., 2011: 146). There are clearly people who try new activities in retirement despite ageing, but the development of a pathology is linked to a significant decrease in leisure activity in general. Burlot and Lefèvre (2010) make similar observations concerning the practice of sport, with sporty seniors becoming more committed upon retirement. On the other hand, they also observe that retirement does not appear to encourage non-sporty people to convert to sport. While it is commonly believed that 'ageing bodies are devoid of any resources whatsoever' (Tulle, 2008: 9), major social inequalities exist in older people's relationship with physical exercise.

The combined effects of ageing and chronic illness are considerably heightened for the most socially underprivileged populations. Participation in cultural practices and sport is unevenly distributed among senior citizens, according to their position in the social structure (Burlot and Lefèvre, 2010; Jones and Higgs, 2013), and in a way that is completely coherent with the distribution of health-related practices (Banks et al., 2003). Blane (2006) has established that people in higher social categories manage health more successfully. Practices are illustrative of common social representations concerning the body, health, social participation and the very idea of prevention (Perrin et al., 2002). While regular physical exercise forms an integral part of the treatment for type 2 diabetes (subject under study in this chapter), prescribing it medically for socially underprivileged ageing people would not appear to produce desired outcomes. Neither providing information on the benefits of regular physical exercise nor pointing people in the direction of a club would appear sufficient to ensure their long-term commitment to exercise (Perrin, 2012; Barth et al., 2014). Innovative programmes have been designed continuously in France since the early 2000s in order to resolve the issue (Terret and Perrin, 2007). They combine therapeutic education with a series of around twenty practical Adapted Physical Activity (APA) sessions intended to develop the patients' relationships with their bodies by creating new sensations and increasing empowerment. They are also designed to develop people's autonomy. By turning physical activity and sport into cultural practices, they aim to develop people's perceptual, motor, relational, cognitive and communication skills. They do so in a co-construction framework, which gives participants a stake in the process and promotes social contacts. In one of France's particularly socially underprivileged regions, these programmes have led to the setting-up of a sports association for the chronically ill, intended to continue the action launched by health measures. It thus becomes particularly interesting to study the 'commitment' process (Becker, 1960), which leads older patients being medically monitored for type 2 diabetes (T2D) to engage regularly in physical exercise that has been adapted for their new 'ageing patient' condition. Commitment to a series of practical APA sessions, initiated by medical recommendation, must initially be accompanied by care and therapeutic education, especially for those who lack social and cultural capital. It is an integral part of the 'illness trajectory' as defined by Anselm Strauss (Strauss et al., 1985: 8), namely in reference to the 'physiological development of the disease, as well as to all efforts undertaken to follow the course taken'. The focus is on a holistic approach to the disease by all participants throughout the course of the illness and on its management. The approach is interesting in that it combines two levels of analysis: that of the participant and that of the various structural constraints, which affect the participant's actions (Corbin and Strauss, 1988). The aim is, therefore, to understand how people progress from their experience of recommended and supervised APA as part of their health care programme to self-determined practice, which finds its own place in their life plan. The paper's focus on ageing adults on lower income gives access to greater understanding about how a population group with a tradition of resisting medical recommendations experiences the APA programme.

In this respect, we will draw upon the concept of 'career', defined by Howard Becker (1985) as being the 'path or progression of a person during his life or a given part of it'. The concept of 'career' makes it possible to identify moments of continuity and discontinuity. At each of these moments, there exists an explanation, which is linked to a necessary behavioural cause. We may therefore imagine this 'career' as being made up of times when the practitioner gives up, starts new activities or has a break, in short a whole series of choices that the practitioner makes with regard to his aims, representations of the activity, possibilities of action, social networks, and so forth. The 'APA practitioner career' refers to the continuous sequential adjustment of an individual to the world of physical activity and sport. Our study will focus particularly on the passage from 'illness trajectory' to 'APA practitioner career', which takes place autonomously in associations and/or which results in a more active 'lifestyle. In other words, how do the new forms of medical care concerning chronic illness succeed in sustaining an unlikely commitment to physical activity? Ultimately the chapter highlights the role played by appropriate educational support for physical activity in overcoming social inequalities among the ageing population without which, we posit, physical activity would merely reinforce these inequalities.

Methods

The study is based on 27 in-depth interviews carried out with 22 type 2 diabetes sufferers who became members of a patients' sports association after completing a therapeutic education programme 'in and via' Adapted Physical Activity. They have co-morbidities and have difficult social conditions (family problems, loneliness, financial problems and so forth). The aim is to reconstruct, over three years, stages in patients' experiences of the disease and the various forms of APA. Following diagnosis of the disease, the 22 interviewees complied with the prescription to engage in APA as part of their care path before deciding to continue the experience in the association. The association called Bouger Pour sa Santé (Get Moving for Health) has several slots in a local gym which members use as their meeting point. It offers a wide range of physical activities (aqua aerobics, gymnastics, basketball, muscle strengthening, walking etc). The objectives expressed go well beyond promoting, starting and continuing physical activity for good health. The study proposes a detailed analysis of the interactions between all care participants throughout the various construction stages of the person's commitment to an 'APA practitioner career' (Barth et al., 2014). To this end, textual data processing software (Prospéro) was used in order to identify more precisely moments of discontinuity and continuity and to validate or not interpretations. This constant to-ing and fro-ing between observed occurrences and singular statements allowed the identification of essential information about experiences of APA and disease from the interviews (Trabal, 2005).

Findings

Analysis of the accounts identified three periods in the commitment process, which show simultaneously a growing quest for autonomy with regard to prescription medication, heightened personal physical awareness and the development of relational networks.

A 'career' entry point positioned on the 'illness trajectory': learning about body techniques and perception of APA effects

While the research participants did not contest the benefits of physical activity for T2D, their commitment to exercise remained unthinkable upon confirmation of the disease. In general, the T2D patient who does not feel even the slightest symptom will not 'comply' with his/her treatment. Patients' 'non-compliance' thus shows a 'gap between the patient's behaviour and medical opinion' (Sandrin-Berthon, 2008). Not only did they feel unconcerned about physical exercise and sport for cultural reasons, they also viewed the former as being intended solely for young people in good health, since it required a level of performance that exceeded their capabilities and failed to provide any positive experience or sensation. Yet, practicing APA among peers brings a new form of sociability and allows the 'acquisition of body techniques, perception of the effects of exercise' (Becker, 1985: 68). The patient is able to observe the immediate impact of physical exercise on his/her blood sugar level, as well as on the development of new capabilities that s/he had, hitherto, tended to minimise:

> I felt better in myself straightaway, and I enjoyed the feeling of wellbeing I had after exercising...It [physical exercise] enables me to reduce the amount of medication. I take, I didn't have to take my evening tablet. (Nicole, 68, retired stock controller, T2D since 1987, APA in 2003)

APA sessions enable practitioners to feel the effects on the body and to realise that the body may be transformed:

> These 20 sessions have shown me that I am still capable of achieving something and that I can keep on going. (Christian, 79, retired accountant, T2D since 1996, Heart condition since 2004, APA in 2004)

The opportunity to reconnect with physical sensations gives meaning to the activity and ensures that adherence is maintained. The interviews highlight a real change in body perception, with greater care and respect for the body. Discussions among patients also made it possible to encourage each person to act upon the disease through his/her own actions. By discovering and then recognising the signs the body gives (fainting, hypoglycemia, increased flexibility and endurance), the patient becomes capable of acting as a real 'sentry' (Pinell, 1992) and of sounding the alarm in the case of physiological problems. Practicing APA is therefore initially inseparable from organised care and therapeutic education within the medical space itself and during the course of the 'illness trajectory'. This new, time-consuming activity becomes possible, even life-saving, when professional activity ceases.

> I think it's the physical activity that has boosted me a bit, being deprived of my job and then having to live with health problems... it's not that easy to build yourself another life; without going to work every day, and then to realise you have a health problem, you end up feeling a bit diminished... If I've managed to get over the worst, I think in a way it's thanks to the association, sport. (Thérèse, 57, unemployed ambulance driver, T2D since 2002, APA in 2005)

While retirement may be considered as a time conducive to commitment or re-commitment to physical exercise (Henaff-Pineau, 2012; Weiss and Bass, 2002), the loss of one's job may likewise be an opportunity to engage in physical activity and overcome the ordeal and offset the 'social sidelining' that may be a consequence of it.

From 'trajectory' to 'APA practitioner career': developing a taste for the effects of exercise

While some people limit their action to care and therefore remain in the 'illness trajectory', the majority of interviewees had developed not only a taste for the effects of exercise, but also became determined to continue physical exercise for the satisfaction they derived from it. This new form of leisure-oriented exercise makes transforming a person's 'lifestyle' a reality, and marks the beginnings of commitment to autonomous and medically unrelated physical activity (Barth et al., 2014). This is what makes association membership possible. Accounts show interviewees' satisfaction with progressing within the association outside of a medical context. The association becomes a new living space (Marcellini, 2010), a place for conviviality and sharing experiences. Members have gone so far as to organise cookery and beauty therapy workshops with the aim of sharing knowledge. Some meet up after APA sessions to attend shows and sometimes even longer events (information days, forums, spas and so forth).

> I usually come for a coffee every Monday, we meet up before the gym lesson and I chat for a bit... it feels good to be surrounded by nice people, and the old girls, well I know I can count on them. (Patricia, 75, Obesity, T2D since 1990, APA in 2002)

As an element of T2D 'triptych care' (with the recommendation of diet and medication), APA is also a tool for expanding individuals' cultural capital, and thus provides a context conducive to extending the social network that is only too often eroded by ageing (Tulle, 2012; Cumming and Henry, 1961).

We help each other, we comfort each other, we share things. When someone doesn't feel too good, we're there for them, we support each other, because we understand the situation, and that, for me, that's important. (Antoine, 67, retired miner, Obesity, T2D since 2002, Heart condition since 2003, APA in 2003)

APA enables patients to gain access to another dimension, where they can enjoy getting together and sharing mutual experiences. Relationships and social interactions are considered to be of utmost importance, so much so that at times they take priority over the physiological benefits of the activity.

I enjoy coming to the association, we have great fun, there's a good atmosphere, it's very important for me, otherwise, I wouldn't come. (Ghislaine, 58, retired teaching assistant, Obesity, T2D since 1997, depression in 1997, APA in 2002)

Through the new sensations it provides and an extended social network, APA becomes a deliberate choice, losing its association with medical prescription. This autonomy is built on the solidarity of experiencing shared ordeals resulting from chronic illness.

Complete conversion to APA

For the minority of interviewees, being in an association ensures regular exercise, which in turn, enables them to build their own individual health norms. Interviewees express a new feeling of being in control with regard to health management, as well as the possibility of modifying further components of their lifestyle. In this case, engaging in the 'APA practitioner career' produces a boomerang effect on the 'illness trajectory'. Contributions confirm the development of new empowerment, including continued investment in disease management through regular intake of medication and a sustained personal resolution to regulate eating habits and use of substances (tobacco, alcohol, stimulants, and so forth). Patients seek to exercise self-control in a self-determined way, 'to identify and satisfy their needs, resolve their problems and call upon personal resources so as to have the feeling of being in control of their own lives' (Gibson, 1991: 355). They assert their status as 'expert' patient, playing an active role in the management of their disease.

I realised I had to act, that I couldn't just do nothing, to start with, it was through sport at the association, now, it's different, I keep an eye on almost everything..., I know what I have to do and how to do it, it concerns a whole lot of different things. (Odile, 60, Concierge, Obesity, T2D since 2000, APA in 2003)

A minority of informants referred to a new form of social participation. Their association experience enabled them to open up to new possibilities, to redefine future prospects as regards the disease and to participate in new activities (self-care, membership in 'ordinary' associations).

As for me, I was willing to ignore my body.... My body just stored it all up, and that's what happened when I had my depression...I couldn't accept that anybody could love me.... My face, eyes, taking care of everything that's just about presentable, I need to do that because it's an important part of my relationships with others, and I use different creams as well now, it's not about trying to be attractive, and it's nothing to do with old age, it's just that I need to do that, I need to stop myself feeling any worse about myself. (Ghislaine, 58, retired teaching assistant, Obesity, T2D since 1997, suffering from depression, APA in 2002).

People's accounts of their experiences highlight their new empowerment with regard to their bodies, in spite of disease and ageing. They express greater confidence in their bodies. They are less concerned about other people's opinions in their daily actions, as well as in those including movement, which in turn contributes to greater self-esteem (Phoenix and Sparkes, 2008). In this respect, the practical experience of exercising holds a decisive place in the 'T2D trajectory' when it comes to the construction of patient autonomy in management of their disease. It is through experiencing and becoming aware of what is right for them that patients suffering from chronic illness decide to implement new norms in the way they live with their illness.

Conclusion

The study provides greater understanding of how older T2D sufferers from middle and working class backgrounds engage in an 'APA practitioner career'. While APA was at first of no concern to them, innovative care measures, which combine APA and therapeutic education (continued and shared experience, peer groups) gave them the opportunity to socialise through physical exercise and body care. By practicing regular physical activity, people with diabetes become experts in their own bodies, manage their disease and plan new projects. Initially considered highly improbable, their commitment to physical exercise gave rise to new reflections on the meaning of 'active ageing'. However, without the necessary educational support to compensate for their social status deficit, this objective runs the risk of reinforcing social inequality and stigmatising those who lack social and financial capital.

The encouragement to engage in active ageing or to 'age well' reflects middle class ideology and privilege, constituting in this way a process of cultural and moral normalisation. Merely conveying the messages of illness prevention campaigns, known to be socially close to the ethos of 'educated' social categories (Génolini and Clément, 2010) is not sufficient to support population groups with low financial and social resources. Given the ineffectiveness of information and recommendation measures being a well-known fact today, should we not turn to a discourse which gives primacy to embodied practices, muscle tone, motor skills, perceptions and emotions, and which recognises the social dimension of cultural practices.

Researching how sick and underprivileged older people develop an APA career highlights the importance of the social experience of physical activity supported over the long term by an experienced APA instructor, whose approach to teaching meets participants' needs, corresponds to their resources and is meaningful to them (Perrin et al., 2008). 22 stories insist on supporting all health professionals in their commitment to physical activity and more generally in changing lifestyles. Professionals' role is to help people develop, over the long term, an APA career, which enables them to play an active role in their own recovery but also to develop forms of social and cultural capital, which would have been denied to them without the APA.

Demedicalised APA becomes established in the social and takes over everyday life. Thus greater well-being, ageing better and living better with the disease can be goals that older people set themselves and negotiate. The aims of public policies are frequently conveyed by institutions to individuals, making the latter responsible for the success of the objectives. These objectives run the risk of becoming normalising moral commands. On the other hand, if they are actively pursued by institutions, organisations and professions in dialogue with the population groups concerned, they can become humanist objectives, and with appropriate professional support, transform the disease experience into an opportunity to fight social inequalities.

References

Banks J, Karlsen S and Oldfield Z (2003) Socio-economic position. In: M Marmot et al. (eds) *Health, Wealth and Lifestyles of the Older Population in England: The 2002 English Longitudinal Study of Ageing.* London: Institute for Fiscal Studies, pp. 71–125.

Barth N, Perrin C and Camy J (2014) S'engager dans une pratique régulière d'activité physique (AP) lorsqu'on est atteint de diabète de type 2: entre «trajectoire de maladie» et «carrière de pratiquant d'Activité physique adaptée». *Loisir et société* 37(2): 224–240.

Becker H (1985) *Outsiders, Etude de la Sociologie de la Déviance* (1st edition 1963). Paris: Métaillé.

Becker H (1960) Notes on the concept of commitment. *American Journal of Sociology* 66: 32–40.

Blane D (2006) The life course, the social gradient, and health. In: M Marmot and RG Wilkinson (eds) *Social Determinants of Health.* Oxford: Oxford University Press, pp. 54–77.

Burlot F and Lefèvre B (2010) Le sport et les séniors: des pratiques spécifiques? *Retraite et Société* 58: 134–158.

Corbin J and Strauss AL (1988) *Unending Work and Care: Managing Chronic Illness at Home.* San Francisco: Jossey-Bass.

Cumming E and Henry WE (1961) *Growing Old: The Process of Disengagement.* New York: Basic.

Feillet R (2000) *Pratiques Sportives et Résistances au Vieillissement.* Paris: L'harmattan.

Génolini JP and Clément JP (2010) Lutter contre la sédentarité : l'incorporation d'une nouvelle morale de l'effort, Laboratoire sport organisation Identités. *Revue Sciences Sociales et Sport* 3: 133–156.

Gibson CH (1991) A concept analysis of empowerment. *Journal of Advanced Nursing* 16: 354–361.

Henaff-Pineau PC (2012) Le senior sportif, une nouvelle figure du bien vieillir? *Les Politiques Sociales* 72(1–2): 101–112.

Henaff-Pineau PC (2009) Vieillissement et pratiques sportives: entre modération et intensification. *Lien Social et Politiques* 62: 71–83.

Jones IR and Higgs PF (2013) Class and health inequality in later life. In: M Formosa and P Higgs (eds) *Social Class in Later Life: Power, Identity and Lifestyle.* Bristol: Policy Press. pp.113–131.

Marcellini A (2010) Les usages du sport par et pour les personnes handicapées. *Sport et Citoyenneté* 12: 17.

Ministère de la santé et des solidarités, *Programme National Nutrition Santé*, PNNS 1 (2001–2005), PNNS 2 (2006–2010), PNNS 3 (2011–2015), Actions et mesures, Recommandations de santé publique. Available at: http//www.mangerbouger.fr/pnns (accessed February 2014).

Ministère de la santé et des solidarités, Plan bien vieillir 2007–2009. Available at: http://travail-emploi.gouv.fr/IMG/pdf/presentationplan-3.pdf (accessed February 2014).

Nicolson L (2004) Older People, Sport and Physical Activity: A Review of Key Issues, Research Report no. 96. Edinburgh: Sport Scotland. Available at: http://www.

sportscotland.org.uk/Documents/Research_Reports/older_people_report_final. pdf (accessed February 2014).
Perrin C (2012) Exercice du patient ou mouvement de la personne malade? L'introduction de l'APA dans le secteur médical confrontée à la valeur d'autonomie. In: B Andrieu (ed) *Ethique du Sport*. Lausanne, Switzerland: Editions l'Age d'Homme, pp 328–339.
Perrin C, Champely S, Chantelat P, Sandrin-Berthon B, Mollet E., Tabard N et al. (2008) Activité Physique Adaptée et Education du Patient dans les Réseaux Diabète Français. *Santé Publique* 3: 213–223.
Perrin C, Ferron C, Gueguen R, et al. (2002) Lifestyle patterns concerning sports and physical activity, and perceptions of health. *International Journal of Public Health*, 47: 162–171.
Phoenix C and Sparkes AC (2008) Athletic bodies and aging in context: the narrative construction of experienced and anticipated selves in time. *Journal of Aging Studies*, 22(3): 211–221.
Pinell P (1992) *Naissance d'un Fléau, Histoire de la Lutte Contre le Cancer en France (1890–1940)*. Paris: Métailié (Leçons de choses).
Poortmans JR and Carpentier YA (2009) Sarcopénie, vieillissement et exercice, Sciences et sport. Available at: http://www.em-consulte.com/article/206973 (accessed February 2014).
Sandrin-Berthon B (2008) L'éducation thérapeutique, pourquoi? *Médecine des Maladies Métaboliques* 2(2): 155–159.
Scherger S, Nazroo J and Higgs P (2011) Leisure activities and retirement: do structures of inequality change in old age? *Ageing and Society* 31: 146–172.
Sparkes AC, Pérez-Samaniego V and Smith B (2012) Social comparison processes, narrative mapping, and their shaping of the cancer experience: a case study of an elite athlete. *Health: An Interdisciplinary Journal for the Study of Health, Illness and Medicine* 5(16): 467–488.
Strauss AL, Fagerhaugh S, Suczeck C and Wiener C (1985) Social organization of Medical work. In: *La Trame de la Négociation: Sociologie Qualitative et Interactionnisme*, textes réunis et présenté par I Baszanger (1992). Paris: L'harmattan, pp. 8–39.
Terret T and Perrin C (2007) Activité physique des personnes atteintes d'un diabète en France: du rejet de la pratique à sa promotion par les associations de patients. *Stadion* 33(2): 185–206.
Trabal P (2005) Le logiciel Prospéro à l'épreuve d'un corpus de résumés sociologiques. *Bulletin de Méthodologie Sociologiques (BMS)* 85: 10–43.
Tulle E and Dorrer N (2012) Back from the brink: ageing, exercise and health in a small gym. *Ageing and Society* 32(7): 1106–1127.
Tulle E (2008) *Ageing, the Body and Social Change: Running in Later Life*. London: Palgrave Macmillan.
Weiss R and Bass S (2002) Introduction. In: R Weiss and S Bass (eds) *Challenges of the Third Age*. Oxford: Oxford University Press, pp 3–12.

6
Pathways to Masters Sport: Sharing Stories from Sport 'Continuers', 'Rekindlers' and 'Late Bloomers'

Rylee A. Dionigi

Introduction

In this chapter I draw from interview data on older athletes (over 75 years old) who regularly compete in individual sports, such as running, swimming, cycling and racquet sports (Dionigi, 2008). I make sense of this data using the work of Jones and Higgs (2010) and Bauman (2000), among others, on normative pronouncements as they relate to ageing, activity, health and fitness in contemporary society. The 7 people who are the focus of this chapter were born between 1913 and 1926. They have experienced The Great Depression, World War I and/or World War II. In addition, they have lived through a cultural period in which understandings of ageing were predominantly associated with the acceptance of natural bodily decline (Jones and Higgs, 2010) and sport was considered inappropriate, dangerous and unnecessary for women and older people (Grant, 2001; Dionigi, 2010). Now older adults live in a climate that is shaped and defined by a resistance to old age and one in which 'active ageing' is promoted in media reports, government policies and in the sport/exercise sciences (Pike, 2011; Tulle, 2008; World Health Organization, 2002).

Since the 'fitness boom' in the 1970s and the emergence of 'successful aging' discourses (for example, Rowe and Kahn, 1997) in the 1980s and 1990s, it has been argued in research and policy that 'old muscles are supposed to be moved' (Grant, 2001: 780). In this climate, sport and physical activity are positioned as crucial in delaying age-related decline and reducing the risk of many chronic conditions (Tulle, 2008). Today everyone is highly encouraged to keep physically, mentally and socially active to maintain their health and, consequently, opportunities to participate in structured physical activity/exercise, such as Masters sport, are readily available.

Theoretical framework

To contextualise this change in understandings and opportunities related to ageing, it is important to consider the shift from modernity to 'second modernity' and the associated construction of the Third and Fourth Ages (Jones and Higgs, 2010). Jones and Higgs, among others, characterise second modernity in terms of individualisation, fragmentation and the 'normalization of diversity' (2010: 1514). That is, since the nineteenth century there has been a shift away from the production-based ideals and prescribed functions of modernity to a focus on consumption, individual choice, leisure and pleasure. As a consequence, understandings of ageing that were the norm during modernity, such as the acceptance of decline and dependency in old age, are 'banished to the margins' in second modernity where the focus is on 'self-care which is aimed at delaying or denying bodily decline (Jones and Higgs, 2010: 1516). This shift has contributed to older people becoming the valued targets of anti-ageing products and services that promote youthfulness and active living under the banner of 'active ageing' (Gilleard and Higgs, 2002, 2000). Masters sport is just one example.

Higgs et al. (2009) argue that these new consumer markets provided the basis for certain generational identities, such as the Third Age, to emerge in the latter half of the twentieth century. A key feature of the Third Age is 'the effective use of leisure' and ongoing engagement in 'activity, exercise, travel, eating out, self-maintenance and self-care' (Gilleard and Higgs, 2007: 25; Laslett, 1989). There is a moral imperative embedded in the desire to remain healthy, active and engaged, as shown in Bauman's (2000: 78) discussions around 'the pursuit of fitness' in contemporary consumer society. A goal of the Third Age is to delay or prevent the Fourth Age, which is characterised by sickness, dependency, frailty and the imminence of death (Blaikie, 1999). Being exposed to these multiple and conflicting discourses and opportunities associated with ageing and activity throughout their lives undoubtedly influenced the way the participants in this chapter rationalised their interest, competitive practices and experiences in physically demanding pursuits.

Sporting backgrounds

The participants include three men and four women who were aged between 76 and 89 during the time of their interview. They were part of a wider qualitative study that involved in-depth interviews with 28 athletes (15 females) aged 60–89 years and participant observations at the 8th Australian Masters Games in Newcastle, Australia (Dionigi, 2008). In-depth interviews were 50–150 minutes in length and focused on sporting history, the role and meaning of sport in their life, current experiences in sport and future plans. All participants detailed in this chapter were white, married or widowed and resided in their own homes in cities across eastern New South Wales, Australia. They competed in the Australian Masters Games (AMG) and were members of a Masters or Veterans' club for their particular sport.

Masters sport (that is, sporting clubs at the local level that run weekly training and competitions) and major multi-sporting events, like the Australian and World Masters Games, are increasing in popularity in post-industrial nations (Weir et al., 2010). The 2005 World Masters Games (WMG) in Edmonton, Canada, had 21,600 registered participants, the 2009 WMG in Sydney had approximately 28,600 competitors, and the 2013 WMG in Italy attracted close to 20,000 participants (www.imga-masters.com). Approximately half of Masters participants are continuers of sport. The other half consists of people who had played sport/were physically active in their youth and then (after a long break) returned to the sporting context to 'rekindle the flame' or who were not 'sporty' and began competing in sport later in life (Dionigi et al., 2013). These trends raise questions about the possible personal and cultural effects of this growing interest in late life sport participation. For example, what are the potential opportunities and difficulties of attempting to maintain fitness and activity in old age and what are the dangers of framing an athletic older age as 'the way' to age?

Specifically, this chapter shares the stories of two sport continuers, two re-starters of sport/physical activity and three late life beginners to sport/physical activity. Among these athletes there is great diversity and complexity in individual pathways to Masters sport as well as commonalities. Two broad areas cutting across the data, that are the focus of discussion, are a typology of pathways (sport 'continuers', 'rekindlers' and 'late bloomers') and the embodiment of 'active ageing'. By locating these athletes' stories in the broader social and political contexts of their time, it is recognised that older people who invest in Masters sport are an exclusive and privileged group (on the basis of class, access, and/

or ability) who do not represent the majority of older people living in Western countries. In addition, discussing these stories in terms of the theoretical conundrum that active ageing presents, such as how discourses on the natural and the normative in relation to ageing (Jones and Higgs, 2010) and the ongoing pursuit of fitness can set up unattainable goals (Bauman, 2000), allows one to appreciate the complexities inherent in the active ageing agenda.

Typology of pathways

Lifelong 'continuers' of sport

The sport continuers, Victoria and Alena, both 76 years old, have been involved in tennis for most of their lives. However, they came from different class backgrounds. Victoria was from a privileged family with a focus on sport, particularly tennis. She was coached in her youth and competed regularly in the city. Victoria has remained committed to tennis since her family migrated from England to Australia shortly after World War I. Not only was sport 'a way of life' for Victoria in her youth, it remained 'vital in [her and her husband's] lives' and it was something that came naturally to her:

> And so consequently, sport all the time, and I think right back when I was a youngster, without knowing it, my mother was encouraging me, like I learnt ballet dancing, I was in physical culture teams, it was sort of, easy to go into it, and I must admit I'm an *extremely* lucky person that I have been able to keep physically fit and enjoy that part without a great deal of effort...I have just enjoyed sport because of that.

Victoria's parents joined an exclusive tennis club 'just after the First World War' which enabled her to start:

> playing comp[etition tennis] with my sister when I was 10...the war had started in 1940 and I was 15...and there was still representative, children's tennis [in my city]...I also played at Sydney University...I played in a team in [a regional inland town in New South Wales] with the air force [during the War]...got married, started to have children, but moved to [a coastal town], tennis was *so strong*, for a *tiny* little town of 2500. We had *five* tennis courts and *so* many played on a Sunday.

58 *Rylee A. Dionigi*

Tennis was clearly a priority in Victoria's life, but it was also always accessible to her and she had a supportive husband who shared childcare responsibilities while she played.

Alternatively, Alena came from a working class background and she was fortunate enough to be given a tennis racquet for making it into a reputable coastal high school. She swam at the beach in her youth and as an older adult she has the convenience (and fortune) of swimming laps in her neighbour's pool every morning (despite the change in home owners). Although Alena did not have the opportunities expressed by Victoria, playing tennis was important to her identity and upbringing:

> [I]n my day there wasn't organised sport, you just grew up on the beach and I think I got a tennis racquet for getting into Newcastle High, that was a *big, big* thing to get your own tennis racquet...But to me it was a way of life. I did play competitive, but there wasn't much during the war years, of course, there were lack of tennis balls, but I still managed to play...because there wasn't much else to do...in the Depression times...so I know what it was like to have nothing.

Like many continuers of sport, these two women clearly had a disposition towards sport and physical activity from a young age. They were both naturally competent in the use of their bodies, and they had family support and opportunities to play, despite their different class backgrounds. The women were expressing a Third Age identity through their maintenance of activity in later life, which highlights that such an understanding of ageing only speaks of and to those who have the means, ability and desire to remain active (Blaikie, 1999; Gilleard and Higgs, 2002, 2000).

'Rekindlers' of sport and physical activity

Marjorie, age 82, and Eldon, age 79, were both physically active in their youth. Marjorie was a runner, and Eldon swam. Although they were not involved in regular training or competitions until they joined a Masters/Veteran's club much later in life, they had always considered themselves competitive and 'good' at their chosen sport. Their reasons for having a break from sport, and later returning to it, were largely gender-based.

Marjorie explains that she became involved in track and field Athletics (as an official, not competitor) when she was aged 42 because her young daughters began competing. Even though she did not start competing in 'Fun Runs' until the age of 60, she identified as a runner with a competitive 'drive' or 'streak' from a young age:

[W]hen I was younger there was no athletics, put it that way, out here, for the girls anyway...we weren't in an area that took in athletics. Well in those days, you only had picnics [for miners who worked in the coal mines]...I always went in races at the picnics. I was always a good runner earlier in life...I was always out to win.

When her daughters had grown up and her father had passed away Majorie restarted running races:

I've always enjoyed running, see, it's been *part* of me. I was always a person I didn't walk, I run, you know [smiles]...I suppose it's just the competitiveness in me is why I do it anyway...I just have a little bit of a laugh at times because, my father was a man that never worried about sport much, he wasn't into sport, as far as women doing sport, I mean, he wasn't interested...and if *he knew* that I could still run, at my age now, [laughs] he'd be *so amazed* it wouldn't be funny.

Marjorie expresses a sense of thrill in terms of challenging gender-appropriate norms and she explained during her interview that she hopes to inspire more women to participate in sport. For many women, competing in sport was about resisting gender norms of the female body as passive and weak and challenging sport as the domain of youth and men (Dionigi, 2010).

Also, many Masters athletes receive active encouragement from their children to remain involved in sport as they age (Dionigi et al., 2012). For example, Marjorie says:

[O]ne of the reasons I compete still, I've got two daughters who push me into it, put it that way, yeah they keep me going. They'll say, 'Come on mum' you know like, 'You can do it' sort of thing...we've always sort of loved sport, the whole lot of us, we've all played, done sport...they encourage me to get going and do everything.

Eldon describes how he was always a swimmer, but he did not begin competing until he joined the Diggers [returned soldiers' club] at age 50 and the Masters when aged in his 70s:

Well when I was a kid I used to swim, I used to do...a lot of rock fishing around Sydney...but I never learnt to swim...Well, you know I just kept on going the way I was...I did a little bit of long distance swimming when I was younger...we were swimming nearly every day when I was involved in [the army]...we used to have to swim out and unload the barge...but then I didn't do any until I joined the Diggers, but now I've started to go in the Masters.

Masters athletes who have returned to sport in mid-life have reported feeling that they had more time and energy to devote to sport participation because of diminishing childcare responsibilities (primarily women) or they were no longer working full-time (Dionigi et al., 2012; Litchfield and Dionigi, 2011).

Some participants would never have contemplated joining Masters sport if it was not for a friend or acquaintance suggesting it to them. For example, Eldon joined the Masters to get a better workout and because he was persuaded by a neighbour. In a study on Masters swimmers, Stevenson (2002: 133) referred to these processes as 'seekership' and 'solicited recruitment' – that is, 'people seek out involvement in an activity in order to satisfy some sort of felt need or because of an attraction'. As Eldon (79 years) explains:

> [A] mate across the road he said, we wanted to do a bit more extra training, because I was getting a bit older and I wanted to do a bit extra...so, [his neighbour] suggested it, joining the Masters, so I said, 'Oh yes, I'll go and join'. So we went down and joined it, but he didn't like the long distance swimming so he pulled out, well I stayed with it, that was about three years ago.

Now Eldon has become immersed in the sub-culture of Master swimming. He keeps records on his computer of his individual swims, his club's points and each club member's points as a hobby. Stevenson (2002: 137) describes this process as:

> conversion to the subculture of masters swimming...the swimmer becomes an insider, and so increasingly values that subculture and becomes ever more embedded into it...the more that one becomes entangled in the everyday affairs of the activity, the deeper one's involvement becomes.

To contextualise this desire to remain active and fit, Bauman (2000) argues that, in a consumer society, the fit body is a healthy and valued body because a fit body can keep consuming (Jones and Higgs, 2010). In contrast, the unfit body is not valued and is positioned as a threat to the market and society. While the pursuit of fitness has become an object of desire, working towards bodily fitness in later life is 'ultimately unachievable in a context that demands that it is continually strived for' (Jones and Higgs, 2010: 1518). I will return to this point in the conclusion section.

'Late bloomers': beginners of sport in old age

The three late-life beginners of sport were Edward (81 years, cycling), Janet (80 years, swimming) and Kenneth (89 years, runner and walker). They were not involved in sport as youths nor were they physically competent. Sport was not encouraged (Janet), not available (Edward) or not an interest (Kenneth) when they were young. Tragic late-life events instigated them to begin sport, such as a health scare or the death of a spouse.

Edward explains why he began cycling at age 66, 'I had a subarachnoid haemorrhage [in the brain]... so it was recovering from that that more or less introduced me to cycling'. Although Edward claims to have remained fit through his work as a builder, he was not competent in sport or physical activity in his youth:

> I had no sport until I was 66 years old, I had no sport. I could not kick a football. I never, ever tried to play hockey, I never, ever tried to run and... like I say, it's something that developed, being a cyclist... but having gone that far [now] I don't want to stop it. I don't want to stop. If I wasn't caring for my wife, I would be going to Russia in July and Austria in August... I've got the ability to do it, in the first place and... I don't have to be driven to it.

He explained that becoming a cyclist 'was just like hosing something in the garden and I just let it bloom and kept going'. At the same time, unlike the majority of older adults in society, Edward had sufficient resources to travel, pay for club membership and tournament entrance fees, afford injury rehabilitation and buy sports equipment (Dionigi, 2008). Like Eldon (re-kindler) in the previous section, Edward explains how he became immersed in the competitive cycling culture and the 'pursuit of fitness' (Bauman, 2000: 78):

> I met up with a chap who was interested in weekend cycling, like going for rides here and there... and somebody says, 'Why don't you race on the bike?' Well you think they're sort of making fun of you, and this is just the way I did take it up and then my son... he got a bike also and we joined the cycling club on the same day [he was 66 years old]... you find out that because you're a member of a club

and because you're going to and be competitive, therefore you want to improve your fitness, you want to eat suitable food, you want to train...and it's fascinating, it's interesting, if you become *involved* in this.

Kenneth began long distance walking at age 81 after his wife passed away. One day he decided to walk from his suburb to the nearest city, which was 34 km away. It took him seven hours, including breaks. He said, 'to get out and do this walk was just a fight back to how I missed her'. For many widows, like Kenneth and Janet, leisure pursuits in later life allow them to experience a renewed sense of self (Kleiber, 1999). Kenneth now walks regularly around his town, he is the oldest member of a local walking club and he competes in Fun Runs. Kenneth keeps records of his times and displays the awards and trophies he has gained from running and walking in a garage under his home:

> I didn't know what the meaning of athlete [as a youth, he was a singer/actor], couldn't run...I didn't think I had any ability on the athletic field. I was always pretty thin, but I've got a good strong pair of legs and it's just since, since my wife died, well I found out that I could walk without any problems, so I thought, "I must be pretty fit."

In contrast to most of the other stories shared in this chapter, Janet is not competitive and does not keep track of her times or train hard, she 'just swim[s]'. Janet began going for walks, gardening, line dancing (and later swimming) during her retirement years:

> I was never ever interested in sport...I used to read...I wasn't sort of an active person growing up. I was a shy, little thing [laughs]. Now I've changed...it was over the Christmas holidays and all of our organisations had stopped, you know there was no garden club, no Probus [a group for retired professionals], no walking group, no, everything had stopped, and I was *bored to tears*... [her future coach] was talking about swimming, you know, he said there was adult learn to swim classes...so I just went round and, it all started from there...And I re[member], when I came out of the pool that morning, I felt *that good* and *invigorated* and I thought, 'Oh this is great!'

Janet is primarily interested in the social element of swimming:

[I]t's the company too, they're all nice people and, they're different friends again [from those at line dancing]...it's the friendship too and the social part of it...I think it keeps you brighter, I mean if you didn't have any friends, you'd be sitting at home. I couldn't do that [starts to laugh] I'm not a sit at home person. I'm out all the time...As I say, if you didn't have any friends and you didn't go out, wouldn't it be a miserable old life?

Social contact, enjoyment and friendships are key reasons why many 'late bloomers' (and re-starters) began sport because most of them are living alone (due to having been widowed, divorced or never married) or caring for an ill spouse (who has dementia or is disabled, for example) (Dionigi, 2008). In addition, Janet's story (like all the stories shared in this chapter) reflects a society that values independence, ability and competitiveness (that is, a Third Ager) and disparages 'other' ways of ageing, such as 'sitting at home' (that is, someone in the Fourth Age). In her final sentence above, Janet is casting a moral judgement that being physically and socially active is a 'good way' or 'the correct way' to age – a finding that is elaborated below.

Embodiment of 'active aging'

When talking about sport and ageing, highly active older people tend to mobilise simplistic notions of what constitutes 'good' and 'bad' ageing that underpin the active ageing agenda. This way of thinking has the potential to reproduce ageism and blame inactivity for disease (or premature death) – possible effects of the Masters sport movement (Dionigi, 2008). For example, later in her interview, Janet explains:

[W]ell, I had a friend...and *all she did* was sit in a lounge chair and watch TV, and she'd say, 'But I can't, I can't walk'...See, she wasn't *active*...it is important to *keep* yourself *active*, even if you just walk around the yard, or just walk up and down the street...*you've got to do it!* And then, of course she died at home – no good.

Likewise, Kenneth (late bloomer, 89 years) says:

Just to sit around...your muscles go...keep going...if I was to sit around...I'd get rusty...like a lot of old people do...they're sitting at home getting around in their pyjamas. I know one fellow...he retired...just given everything away...he didn't last very long.

These quotes imply that there is something wrong with sitting around. What if people enjoy the tranquillity of home-life? Some people might look forward to being idle and alone, but in the current discourse, these are not acceptable aspirations for old age (Bauman, 2000; Gilleard and Higgs, 2000, 2002; Jones and Higgs, 2010).

There was also an understanding among the participants that how you age is primarily a matter of choice. This way of thinking ignores social constraints and inequities (as well as the inevitability of physical decline in old age and uncontrollability of most diseases) and further marginalises those who do not have the means, desire or ability to be active or 'get out of their house' (that is, the Fourth Ager). It positions older adults who do not engage in physical activity as lazy, immoral or a burden on society, and those who keep active and remain independent as 'moral citizens' who are doing their duty for society (Katz, 2000). Evidently, there was a strong desire among the participants to remain fit and healthy through sport:

> [B]eing fit as long as you can is perhaps the most *important thing in life*...if you *stop*, you don't get it back, you know, you've just got to keep it going as long as you can and at the ability that you've got, so I think I've been very blessed because of it. (Alena, continuer, 76)

Alongside this appropriation of the health and fitness imperative was an expressed fear of not being able to move, of being ill in old age and of being forced to sit or live in a nursing home. Marjorie explained 'I'd *hate* to think I can't move around, it's distress me to think I couldn't and if I can make myself do it, I'll make myself do it' (rekindler, 82). When asked, 'What does it mean to you to be still playing sport at this point in your life?' Victoria (continuer, 76) replied:

> Making these latter years as enjoyable as I can, by being fit and I do feel that's important because I have a friend I see...who's in a nursing home...This woman is 85 and I know through her what it is like to be in a home and I say to my husband, 'Where is the nearest *gap*? We shall jump over it [commit suicide]', rather than do that [live in a home]. It's like an imprisonment, she feels it, it's morbid, it's sad, it's unfeeling.

In a society that only values ability, competitiveness, consumerism and youthfulness, older people who are independent, highly active and visible receive social recognition and express feelings of self-pride. In such contexts, 'the incapacitated elderly are excluded or abandoned in a clear power struggle' (Mendes, 2013: 177). By way of example, take Kenneth's story (late bloomer, 89). Since Kenneth began going for long walks he has become well-known in his local area and he gets quite a lot of media attention. When asked about being labelled 'a local hero' [one of the headlines in a newspaper article about his walking], he said:

> Oh well, it just proves something to me that... I did have some athletic tendency... It's just proof that I wasn't just a skinny kid... And, you know, it's such a thrill to, if you have people pulling up in the street every day... some that I hardly know... and say, 'Are you still running?' I've achieved something. I'm not such *a weakling*, as I should be... I've *always* thought of that [the time when at age 15 he was offered assistance in a swimming pool because another boy thought he was 'a cripple']. I wonder what that bloke would say, thinking I was a *cripple*, and here *I* am winning age races, I've *found* the one *thing* that I could do on the athletic field.

How will Kenneth cope when the realities of physiological ageing take their toll and he can no longer walk? Will he self-label as 'a weakling' or 'a cripple'? Will society value him then? Is the active ageing agenda creating a generation of people who identify themselves through physical competency and therefore may not be able to mentally cope with ill health and disability in old age? More broadly, how does sport participation in later life allow all of us to think about ageing in our society? To begin to address these questions, below I locate these findings in the context of the theoretical and political conundrum that active ageing presents.

Conclusion

The stories presented in this chapter highlight the contingency (at times pure luck) of not only embarking on a sporting career, but also of having the ability, support, access and structural resources to maintain it over a substantial period of time. The talk of the interviewees illustrates how these people embody the 'active ageing agenda' by simultaneously expressing a fear of not being able to move/being forced to sit/ the nursing home, a negative view of old age, as well as an appropriation of the health and fitness imperative. Since the 1990s 'active ageing' policies, which reflect the current push for older people to 'get out of the house' and 'get off the couch' to remain active and productive in society, have become more prominent in the media and documents associated with social policies for the aged (Mendes, 2013; Pike, 2011). This 'active ageing agenda' is problematic because it emphasises self-responsibility for health, regardless of age, gender, race or social circumstance, and a moral viewpoint is constructed through bipolar conceptions of 'good' and 'bad' ways to age (Pike, 2011). It can perpetuate individual and cultural fear of ill health in old age (Dionigi, 2008) and position exercise in old age as an anti-ageing project, or a form of ageism, rather than as a celebration of ageing in all its forms (Tulle, 2008).

What was particularly evident throughout this chapter was that despite their different pathways to, and when they began, Masters sport, each participant was caught up in the pursuit of health and fitness and desperately attempting to delay or deny the Fourth Age. Although they were all born and raised in a period of modernity, where the norm was to accept bodily decline in old age, they spent their adulthood onwards in a time of plurality and individualisation (Jones and Higgs, 2010). In a contemporary consumer context, that is, 'in a society of infinite and indefinite possibilities' (Bauman, 2000: 79) life is no longer 'normatively regulated', instead it is 'guided by seduction, ever rising desires and volatile wishes' (2000: 76). In discussing the differences between the two terms fitness and health, Bauman explains: 'Unlike the care for health [that, in principle, can be defined and measured], the pursuit of fitness has therefore no natural end' (2000: 78). He adds, in a context of pluralism and fragmentation, 'health-care, contrary to its nature, becomes uncannily similar to the pursuit of fitness: continual, never likely to bring full satisfaction ... and generating on its way a lot of anxiety' (2000: 79). In other words, what it means to be fit or healthy is in a constant state of flux and the desire to be fit or healthy is 'the state of perpetual self-scrutiny' (Bauman, 2000: 78).

Therefore, potential risks of framing highly active older adults as the ideal (under the 'active ageing' banner) include disparaging other ways of ageing, blaming disease on individual inactivity and stigmatising non-participation in sport or activity. While participation in sport (and health promotion in general) is a laudable goal, caution is necessary due to the many personal, cultural and historical factors affecting older adults' inclusion. More critical sport research is needed that starts from the perspectives of a diverse range of older adults, rather than an analysis of how older people's physical activity 'meets' current policy definitions of active ageing that construct physical activity as unanimously worthwhile for all (Aberdeen and Bye, 2013).

References

Aberdeen L and Bye L (2013) Challenges for Australian sociology: critical ageing research ageing well? *Journal of Sociology* 49(1): 3–21.
Bauman Z (2000) *Liquid Modernity*. Cambridge: Polity Press.
Blaikie A (1999) *Ageing and Popular Culture*. Cambridge: Cambridge University Press.
Dionigi RA (2008) *Competing for Life: Older People, Sport and Ageing*. Saarbrücken, Germany: Verlag Dr. Müller.
Dionigi RA (2010) Older sportswomen: personal and cultural meanings of resistance and conformity. *International Journal of Interdisciplinary Social Sciences* 5(4): 395–407.
Dionigi RA, Fraser-Thomas J and Logan J (2012) The nature of family influences on sport participation in Masters athletes. *Annals of Leisure Research* 15(4): 366–388.
Dionigi RA, Horton S and Baker J (2013) Negotiations of the ageing process: older adults stories of sports participation. *Sport, Education and Society* 18(3): 370–387.
Gilleard CJ and Higgs PF (2007) The third age and the baby boomers: two approaches to the social structuring of later life. *International Journal of Ageing and Later Life* 2(2): 13–30.
Gilleard CJ and Higgs PF (2000) *Cultures of Ageing: Self, Citizen, and the Body*. Harlow, UK: Prentice Hall.
Gilleard CJ and Higgs PF (2002) The third age: class, cohort or generation? *Ageing and Society* 22(3): 369–382.
Grant BC (2001) 'You're never too old': beliefs about physical activity and playing sport in later life. *Ageing and Society* 21(6): 777–798.
Higgs PF, Hyde M, Gilleard CJ, Victor CR, Wiggins RD and Jones IR (2009) From passive to active consumers? Later life consumption in the UK from 1968–2005. *Sociological Review* 57(1): 102–124.
Jones IR and Higgs PF (2010) The natural, the normal and the normative: contested terrains in ageing and old age. *Social Science and Medicine* 71(8): 1513–1519.
Katz S (2000) Busy bodies: activity, aging, and the management of everyday life. *Journal of Aging Studies* 14(2): 135–152.
Kleiber DA (1999) *Leisure Experience and Human Development: A Dialectical Interpretation*. New York: Basic Books.
Laslett P (1989) *A Fresh Map of Life: The Emergence of the Third Age*. London: Weidenfeld & Nicolson.
Litchfield C and Dionigi RA (2011) The meaning of sports participation in the lives of middle-aged and older women. *International Journal of Interdisciplinary Social Sciences* 6(5): 21–36.
Mendes FR (2013) Active ageing: a right or a duty? *Health Sociology Review* 22(2): 174–185.
Pike ECJ (2011) The active aging agenda, old folk devils and a new moral panic. *Sociology of Sport Journal* 28(2): 209–225.
Rowe JW and Kahn RL (1997) Successful aging. *The Gerontologist* 37(4): 433–440.
Stevenson CL (2002) Seeking identities: towards an understanding of the athletic careers of Masters swimmers. *International Review for the Sociology of Sport* 37(2): 131–146.

Tulle E (2008) Acting your age? Sports science and the ageing body. *Journal of Aging Studies* 22(4): 340–347.

Weir PL, Baker J and Horton S (2010) The emergence of Masters sport: participatory trends and historical developments. In: J Baker, S Hortonand PL Weir (eds) *The Masters Athlete: Understanding the Role of Sport and Exercise in Optimizing Aging*. London: Routledge, pp. 7–14.

World Health Organization (2002) Active ageing: a policy framework. Available at: http://www.who.int/ageing/publications/active_ageing/en/ (accessed October 2014).

7
Keeping It in the Family: The Generational Transmission of Physical Activity

Victoria J. Palmer

Introduction

The role that family plays in Physical Activity (PA) practices is often overlooked in the PA literature. Nevertheless, family is often identified as a determinant of PA (Bauman et al., 2012; Sherwood and Jeffrey, 2000). Additionally, research into the role that family plays in PA practices tends to focus on children and their parents, rather than how the family may influence PA throughout the life course. Thus, very little is known about how family can impact the PA of older adults or how older adults can influence their families' PA. Therefore, unpacking the role that family plays in PA choices throughout the life course may allow us further insights into the way PA beliefs, understandings and practices are formed, maintained and embodied.

The concept of family is complex, with its own power relations. Families are socially constructed by those within them and the roles and relationships practiced within and by families are influenced by wider social relationships such as gender, class and age (McKie, 2006). The family may be viewed as a key site for socialisation, habitus formation and social reproduction (Bourdieu, 1977). Birchwood et al. (2008) note that the cultural influence of the family is key to the creation of dispositions (habitus) towards sport (or physically active practices) beginning in early childhood. They also suggest that these dispositions can continue to shape PA in adult life. Similarly, Bourdieu (1977) identifies that habitus is first created in the family, aligned with social location and reinforced or changed through interactions with other social structures. Thus, habitus is malleable in nature and there is a constant (re)negotiation of habitus throughout our lives (Dumas and Laberge, 2005). Since we negotiate habitus through interactions and experiences (Bourdieu, 1977), it can be affected by factors such as gender and age. In fact, Tulle (2007) argues that age is just as important as social class in shaping our dispositions and social location through an 'age habitus'. And, although most socialisation occurs during childhood, as we age the family continues 'to shape and contextualise particular aged identities across the life course of its members' (Hockey and James, 2003: 158).

Given the focus on the role of family in children's PA (see Quarmby and Dagkas, 2010; Quarmby et al., 2010; Macdonald et al., 2004), very little is known about how the family can influence PA throughout adulthood and into old age. Some studies have recognised that family can both support and inhibit older adults' PA practices (Dionigi et al., 2012; Young and Medic, 2011). As Tulle (2008a, 2008b) notes, negotiating a PA career can often be at odds with familial obligations, particularly for women. On the other hand, older adults have noted how support from family members has allowed them to continue with PA pursuits (Dionigi et al., 2012). The aim of this chapter, therefore, is to examine older adults' experiences of PA and ageing within the context of the family. It will explore how PA is negotiated in relation to current discourses of PA, health and ageing and the role the family plays in shaping these experiences. Finally it will examine how older adults' PA may influence the younger generations within families and contribute towards familial dispositions towards PA.

Older adults and physical activity

In the latter half of the twentieth century we have seen a surge of research that is informed by sport and exercise science examining the health benefits of PA. However, this prominent body of literature is embedded in narratives of decline, disease and dysfunction and is indicative of a 'moral panic' that surrounds PA and ageing (Pike, 2011). There is an increasing body of work that explores the lived experiences of PA in older adults (see Kluge, 2002; Bundon et al., 2011; Dionigi, 2002; Tulle and Dorrer, 2012), that aims to capture how older adults attribute value and meaning to PA and to illustrate the ways in which older adults engage with discourses of health and ageing (Griffin and Phoenix, 2014). Such studies highlight the complexities of negotiating PA throughout the life course. They also offer an alternative narrative to those of decline and disease that are so prominent in the sport and exercise science literature, noting that for many older adults, PA is empowering; it challenges, resists and redefines understandings of ageing (Dionigi et al., 2013). This research aims to build on these understandings of older adults' PA using the family as a lens to view how older adults negotiate PA and ageing. We can therefore begin to explore the role that family may play in shaping PA throughout the life course.

Background to research

The following findings are part of a larger research project examining PA in three- generational families. The analysis presented here draws upon interview data from two families from the West of Scotland. The families, the Hutchisons and the McDonalds, are from aspiring middle class backgrounds and all the participants self-identified as active. At least one child, one parent and one grandparent from each family participated in the research. Table 7.1 outlines the participating family members for each family. I will focus on the experiences of the grandparents: Donald Hutchison (68) and Elaine McDonald (62). They represent two very different experiences of ageing in relation to their PA that begin to highlight how cultures of PA are created and embodied throughout the life course.

Grandparents' experiences of ageing and physical Activity.

Donald's (68) experience of PA is very much embedded in discourses of health and mirrors traditional narratives of ageing. He had been active throughout his childhood and as a young adult, participating in a variety of sports. In adulthood, his PA declined, becoming irregular and he described is current PA as 'almost non-existent'. The primary reason for this was that he had recently been diagnosed with angina and suffered from arthritis. He had been referred to a cardiac rehabilitation exercise class and had intentions of increasing his PA beyond the

Table 7.1 Description of participants from the Hutchison and McDonald families

	The Hutchison Family	The McDonald Family
Grandparent	Donald (male, 68)	Elaine (female, 62)
Parent	Stuart (male, 34)	Alison (female, 40)
Child(ren)	Aimee (female, 10)	Cara (female, 11)
		Kieran (male, 15)
		Stephanie (female, 18)

cardiac rehabilitation classes (although his practices may not necessarily have reflected this). This kind of reactive behaviour change often occurs following major health changes (Lawton, 2002). At this point in his life, being active was central to improving his health, he stresses 'that's the kind of main factor [affecting PA participation] is looking after my health [sic]'. In addition, he spoke of his ageing body in relation to PA echoing the 'use it or lose' it narratives that others have observed in older adults:

> there is a kind of eh...I was going to say desire but maybe it realisation's maybe a better word that I *need* to do something or the body's just going to give up on me, so eh yip[...]Exercise or start pushing up the daisies [laughs].

Donald returned to PA because of his poor health, although his conditions made PA difficult, noting:

> I'm finding [cardiac rehabilitation classes] very tough, being overweight doesn't help but eh with the arthritis in the joints and that is a painful experience.

PA is often constructed as a moral practice (Dallaire et al., 2012), and as such, not maintaining PA may then be viewed as failing to take responsibility for one's health (Lupton, 1997). For Donald, PA then became a site of moral conflict: he felt he 'needs' to be active, yet his morbidities did not always allow him to act on his intentions. Thus he viewed PA guidelines as unachievable. Since Donald's PA was prescribed by healthcare professionals, we cannot discount that they played a role in the shift towards practicing PA for health, in particular, the cardiac rehabilitation provided Donald with 'expert' information about PA and its benefits to health. The reliance on 'expert' scientific knowledge is prominent in PA policy and can be viewed as a means to normalise PA and prompt people to be active (Dallaire et al., 2012), further contributing to the moralisation of PA.

On the other hand, Elaine (62) continues to be 'regularly active', one of the most active participants in the research. Unlike Donald (68), her activity has been constant throughout her life. To some extent, her experience is perhaps aligned with master athletes who are seen as challenging traditional narratives of ageing (Dionigi, 2002) associated with slowing down. She spoke of such expectations that were expressed by friends and relatives and her resistance to these:

> I think sometimes they [friends] think I'm a wee bit [gestures] daft or something always rushing about and say 'slow down slow down' but if I slow down I'll never get there so I've got to keep going [laughs].

She expresses her desire to keep going, stressing that if she slowed down she'd be 'finished'. Thus she articulates her desire to continue being active into her 'old' age:

> I'd still like to be able to get my at least a walk everyday like you know even when I'm...old [laughs] I'm not old yet [laughs].

Her perception of herself as 'not old' may be an example of how Elaine (62) distances herself from common narratives of ageing. This kind of distancing from ageing stereotypes is not uncommon, particularly for those whose experiences of ageing are active, independent and healthy (Hurd, 1999). However Elaine recognises that ageing has affected her PA in some sense:

> I don't think of myself as being less active now, but I probably was more active then [when she was younger] like you know as I say I still like to do the same things I did then, but probably just take longer [now].

In Tulle's (2007) research with master runners she noted a similar tension. Unlike master athletes, Elaine's PA is not framed as 'leisure' activity. Nor does she train or compete. Instead, her PA, predominantly walking, is practical and functional. In addition, she is not active primarily for health. Contrasting Donald (68), Elaine (62) considers herself to be healthy citing 'aches and pains' as her only ailments. Health, however, was not absent from her PA. She noted that if she is feeling down or tired, walking makes her feel better. Additionally, she identifies that walking functions as a tool for fitness:

> walking gets me from A to B as well as keeping well reasonably fit I could do with losing weight like, but all this walking doesn't seem to do that for me.

But these health benefits are secondary to the functional aspect of walking. Note that she also refers to the need to lose weight. For women, PA is often related to the quest for the 'ideal' fit, slender body (Carlisle Duncan, 2007) and this continues to be relevant, perhaps even more so, for older women whose bodies are often measured in comparison with youthful ideas of beauty (Hurd, 1999). Interestingly, Donald (68) also discusses a need to lose weight, though in his case it is clear that this was directly linked to his recovery from illness.

Familial influence

Both of the grandparents' experiences of PA and ageing were influenced, in some capacity, by their families. In both families, being active was viewed positively, and as a result the grandparents were supported in their PA pursuits. The differences in their experiences of ageing and PA meant that support or encouragement was once again different for each of these grandparents.

For Donald (68), his health was the primary concern of his family, particularly his son (Stuart Hutchison, 34). As a result, Stuart acts as a PA promoter towards his father. Interestingly, this is a role that Stuart also takes with his children. In this sense Stuart (34) engages with current health messages relating to PA, and pro-actively imparts this knowledge to both his children and his father. However, his approach is more subtle towards his father. It takes the form of a 'gentle nudge' highlighted by Donald (68) 'from Stuart I'm getting "oh you'll be able to do a bit of walking when you're away this week" you know? Eh, Nice and gentle but what he's really saying is "you need to do a bit more exercise dad"'. This 'gentle nudge' indicates that there may be some *upward* transmission of PA beliefs understandings and practices.

In the McDonald family, there is a general acceptance of Elaine's (62) activeness, noted mostly by the other family members. For example, her granddaughter Stephanie (18) notes 'my nana, like she's actually like...the fittest person I know'. However, Elaine (62) notes that she has had some negative comments from family members who have told her 'you need to slow down take it easy', in echo of cultural expectations of ageing noted earlier. Despite these occasional comments, her family are generally supportive of, even admiring of her PA. What is also noticeable is that Elaine (62) finds motivation to be active within the family, most notably through her younger grandchildren:

VP: Do you think that your grandchildren's PA influences yours now?

Elaine: It does because I like to be able to keep myself fit so that I can still keep up with them like you know [...] Don't want to be lagging behind them [laughs] sitting in the park saying no I can't play football I'm too old [laughs].

As we are living longer, we've seen a rise in the number of living generations within families, increasing the number of 'years of shared lives' and altering intergenerational dynamics within families (Bengston, 2001). Outwith the family context, intergenerational PA programming is often used as a technique to engage older adults in PA. In the family context, Phoenix and Sparkes (2006) showed that young people drew on older relatives' experiences of ageing and PA to shape their own perceptions of ageing. In this case, Elaine uses her grandchildren to shape her PA, highlighting the importance of intergenerational relationships within families.

Grandparents' role in the family cultures of physical activity

As well as their own experiences of PA being influenced by their families, the grandparents also played a role in creating family cultures of PA. Family cultures of PA reflect shared beliefs, understandings and practices of PA across generations within families. These cultures within families emerge through shared dispositions, and can be influenced by transmission of capitals (social, economic and symbolic) across generations. The Hutchison and McDonald families had particularly clear family cultures of PA although these were manifested in different ways.

The Hutchison family are a 'sporty' family. Their experiences of PA were for the most part related to sport and structured activities. They all had similar experiences of playing sport at school and while the adults' PA participation had declined over the years, these early experiences clearly impacted their current PA choices. Their PA was surrounded by discourses of sport and fitness. They all spoke of achieving fitness (although for Donald this was in relation to his previous activity) and often described their activities using scientific terms such as 'aerobic' or 'cardiovascular'. Moreover, the younger generations engaged with health promotion messages surrounding PA, once again highlighting the role of expert or scientific knowledge in promoting PA.

The McDonalds are 'walkers' and their family culture of PA is visible in their practices. All of the participants in this family walked, and coincidentally they were the most active participating family. What is interesting about this family was that walking held different meanings for the adults and children. Unlike their mother and grandmother, the children did not appear to count walking as PA; they tended to refer to structured activities that they took part in. However, it became clear that all of the children in the family walked to and from school or university and often to the venues of their structured activities. This lack of association of walking with PA in the children may be due to the fact that walking has become embedded in this family's practices (they are predisposed to walking as a constituent part of their habitus). However, it may also reflect changing definitions, understandings and expectations of PA, particularly as the children all participate in 'leisure' activities.

Shaping dispositions

In order to understand how grandparents contribute to family cultures of PA, it is important to consider the changing nature of PA. PA as a health-related behaviour has emerged in recent years, thus it is not surprising that grandparents' understandings of PA were not the same as younger family members. While both grandparents' understandings of PA were related to PA historically, I will use Donald's (68) experiences to illustrate how it can impact family cultures of PA. In the following extract Donald (68) talks about his PA when he was younger:

> When I was a teenager I was exceptionally fit, I was really strong and very flexible and eh...well I mean I could run ten miles that kind of thing, I grew up in the country so I was quite used to throwing around bales of hay and straw and catching recalcitrant sheep and what not and they're quite strong [laughs] [...] eh you'll no remember it but Charles Atlas was around at the time his "Dynamic Tension", I [...] built up a smashing set of muscles including the six pack, I could do 100 press ups and that was fine no problem, eh so then I was really fit I was cycling a lot during the summer I could do 100 miles in a week, [...] eh I swam, I was in the school rugby team, I played cricket, I was in the athletics team, I was exceptionally fit then.

There are several insights into Donald's PA that are illustrated in this statement. Firstly, he describes two different types of PA: functional PA in his duties on the farm and PA for leisure. The distinction between the two types of activity coincides with the emergence of fitness as an act of leisure and as a consumer industry in the latter half of the twentieth century (Smith Maguire, 2002). What is particularly interesting is the way that the activities are framed as he talks about 'being fit' and uses examples to highlight exactly what that means he 'could run 10 miles' and had 'a smashing set of muscles'. What he describes is a particular idea of fitness, one that is embedded in discourses of masculinity that would have been prevalent during his youth. And this discourse can be seen in the way that his family approach PA as sport and structure activities primarily for achieving fitness.

Intergenerational transmission

The other family members realised that the grandparents played a role in shaping their PA beliefs, understandings and practices. In the Hutchison family, Donald's son (Stuart, 34) points out that 'In the family I think there is generally a positive view of exercise and PA'. He talks about how his own attitudes towards PA were shaped by his parents through the opportunities they provided for him to be active, as well as their continued support of his PA. Furthermore, he discusses how he is trying to impart similar beliefs and attitudes to his children 'I think I was fortunate that I had a lot of opportunities [for PA] and that's kind of shaped my attitudes to PA em and I'm hoping that that's coming over for them [his children]'.

In the McDonald family, the intergenerational influences of PA are much more related to practices than beliefs. There is a sense that Elaine's practices are influential, particularly for her daughter and granddaughters. Stephanie (18) notes 'my mum's a pure like walk freak, she walks absolutely everywhere and so does my nana [Grandmother – Elaine] obviously when I was a kid I used to get made to walk it wasn't a choice' and similarly Cara (11) talks about her mother and grandmother when discussing parental influence:

VP: Do you think that your parents' PA influences your PA?
Cara: Em yeah kind of like my mum like walks quite walks quite a lot so like if I was going somewhere my mum would always usually walk [...]
VP: And do you think your grandparents' had any influence on your PA?
Cara: Em the same my nana walked quite a lot so if I was going anywhere with her we'd just walk [...].

The girls talk about walking in a rather nonchalant manner, thus suggesting that walking is so embedded in their lives it is almost second nature. The girls' mother (Alison, 40) also alludes to the influence that her own mother's walking has had on her. Interestingly, Elaine's grandson Kieran (15), the only male participant in the McDonald family, did not view his grandmother's (or mother's) PA as influential. However, he does recognise that his father has influenced his PA, which may suggest that transmission of PA beliefs, understandings and practices is gendered.

Discussion

Using the family as a lens to explore PA offers an opportunity to reveal how people locate PA in their lives, how they negotiate maintaining PA practices and how they may use PA to position themselves in society. The snapshots of PA observed here highlight the complexities of managing PA in our everyday lives. By examining PA across three generations, we gain a unique insight into experiences of ageing and PA in the context of family life. The Hutchison and McDonald families indicate that there may be cultures of PA that emerge within families through shared beliefs, understandings and practices. However, it is also clear that these cultures of PA are influenced by factors beyond the family, including beliefs about, and experiences of, ageing.

It is worth noting that these families' experiences are not indicative of every family. These are two, active, aspiring middle class families from the West of Scotland. The families were 'traditional' in that the grandparents and parents were married or in a long term relationship and the children all lived with both parents. It is likely that families from different class, family and PA backgrounds would have very different experiences of PA (Kay, 2004).

The grandparents had very different experiences of PA and ageing, highlighting the complex nature of negotiating PA throughout the life course. Both experiences were, however, shaped by lifelong dispositions and practices of PA. Others have shown that older adults with lifelong dispositions and practices of PA are more likely to maintain PA as they age, even when faced with barriers such as poor health or disability (Bundon et al., 2011). Their experiences also highlight the centrality of health for older adults' PA, as a prevention or treatment for ill health and as a by-product of being active. The prevalence of health is perhaps unsurprising given its prominence in the sport and exercise science and health promotion literature. Moreover, the grandparents' experiences indicate some of the ways that family can influence how older adults negotiate PA in relation to ageing and health.

Previously, family members have been shown to both support and constrain older adults' PA practices (Dionigi et al., 2012; Young and Medic, 2011). In this instance, family members were largely supportive of PA practices. Additionally, the importance of intergenerational relationships also appeared to influence the grandparents' PA. What is perhaps most notable about these grandparents is the contribution they make to family cultures of PA. The shared beliefs, understandings and practices within these families indicate that dispositions towards PA are created within families, operating throughout the life course – a familial habitus. However, there were also some clear intergenerational differences. It was apparent that age related expectations of PA, as well as experiences of ageing, impacted understandings and practices of PA. This research highlights that family plays a continuous role in shaping dispositions towards PA throughout the life course, albeit in complex ways. However, it also highlights the influence of wider social structures on PA, which together have particular implications for how we understand and promote PA.

References

Bauman AE, Reis RS, Sallis JF et al. (2012) Correlates of physical activity: why are some people physically active and others not? *The Lancet* 380(9838): 258–271.

Bengtson VL (2001) Beyond the nuclear family: the increasing importance of multigenerational bonds. *Journal of Marriage and Family* 63(1): 1–16.

Birchwood D, Roberts K and Pollock G (2008) Explaining differences in sport participation rates among young adults: evidence from the South Caucasus. *European Physical Education Review* 14(3): 283–298.

Bourdieu P (1977) *Outline of a Theory of Practice*. Cambridge: Cambridge University Press.

Bundon A, Clarke LH and Miller WC (2011) Frail older adults and patterns of exercise engagement: understanding exercise behaviours as a means of maintaining continuity of self. *Qualitative Research in Sport, Exercise and Health* 3(1): 33–47.

Carlisle Duncan M (2007) Bodies in motion: the sociology of physical activity. *Quest* 59(1): 55–66.

Dallaire C, Gibbs L, Lemyre L and Krewski D (2012) The gap between knowing and doing: how Canadians understand physical activity as a health promotion strategy. *Sociology of Sport Journal* 29(3): 325–347.

Dionigi R (2002) Leisure and identity management in later life: understanding competitive sport participation among older adults. *World Leisure Journal* 44(3): 4–15.

Dionigi RA, Fraser-Thomas J and Logan J (2012) The nature of family influences on sport participation in Masters athletes. *Annals of Leisure Research* 15(4): 366–388.

Dionigi RA, Horton S and Baker J (2013) Negotiations of the ageing process: older adults' stories of sports participation. *Sport, Education and Society* 18(3): 370–387.

Dumas A and Laberge S (2005) Social class and ageing bodies: understanding physical activity in later life. *Social Theory and Health* 3(3): 183–205.

Griffin M and Phoenix C (2014) Learning to run from narrative foreclosure: one woman's story of aging and physical activity. *Journal of Aging and Physical Activity* 22(3): 393–404.

Hockey J and James A (2003) *Social Identities across the Life Course*. London: Palgrave Macmillan. Available at: http://www.gcu.ac.uk/library/ (accessed June 2014).

Hurd Clarke L (1999) 'We're not old!': older women's negotiation of aging and oldness. *Journal of Aging Studies* 13(4): 419–439.

Kay T (2004) The family factor in sport: a review of family factors affecting sports participation. In: N Rowe (ed) *Driving up Participation: The Challenge for Sport*. London: Sport England.

Kluge MA (2002) Understanding the essence of a physically active lifestyle: a phenomenological study of women 65 and older. *Journal of Aging and Physical Activity* 10: 4–27.

Lawton J (2002) Colonising the future: temporal perceptions and health-relevant behaviours across the adult lifecourse. *Sociology of Health and Illness* 24(6): 714–733.

Lupton D (1997) *The imperative of health: public health and the regulated body*. London: Sage.

Macdonald D, Rodger S, Ziviani J, Jenkins D, Batch J and Jones J. (2004) Physical activity as a dimension of family life for lower primary school children. *Sport, Education and Society* 9(3): 307–325.

McKie L (2006) *Families, Violence and Social Change*. Maidenhead, UK: Open University Press.

Phoenix C and Sparkes AC (2006) Keeping it in the family: narrative maps of ageing and young athletes' perceptions of their futures. *Ageing and Society* 26(4): 631–648.

Pike ECJ (2011) The active aging agenda, old folk devils and a new moral panic. *Sociology of Sport Journal* 32(2): 209–225.

Quarmby T, Dagkas S and Bridge M (2010) Associations between children's physical activities, sedentary behaviours and family structure: a sequential mixed methods approach. *Health Education Research* 26(1): 63–76.

Quarmby T and Dagkas S (2010) Children's engagement in leisure time physical activity: exploring family structure as a determinant. *Leisure Studies* 29(1): 53–66.

Sherwood NE and Jeffery RW (2000) The behavioural determinants of exercise: implications for physical activity interventions. *Annual Review of Nutrition* 20(1): 21–44.

Smith Maguire J (2002) Body lessons: fitness publishing and the cultural production of the fitness consumer. *International Review for the Sociology of Sport* 37(3–4): 449–464.

Tulle E (2007) Running to run: embodiment, structure and agency amongst veteran elite runners. *Sociology* 41(2): 329–346.

Tulle E (2008a) *Ageing, the Body and Social Change: Running in Later Life*. Basingstoke: Palgrave.

Tulle E (2008b) Acting your age? sports science and the ageing body. *Journal of Aging Studies* 22(4) 340–347.

Tulle E and Dorrer N (2012) Back from the brink: ageing, exercise and health in a small gym. *Ageing and Society* 32(7): 1106–1127.

Young BW and Medic N (2011) Examining social influences on the sport commitment of Masters swimmers. *Psychology of Sport and Exercise* 12(2): 168–175.

8
Physical Activity Programmes in Residential Care Settings

Mary Ann Kluge

Background

Residential communities or care settings for older adults are called many things: residential-care communities (RCCs), care centres (CCs), continuing-care retirement communities (CCRCs), or long-term care (LTC) facilities. Distinct from day centres, senior centres, or hospital settings, the popularity of these residential communities varies globally (Dupuis et al., 2012; Iwarsson et al., 2007). Anywhere from 4% to 10% of older U.S. and Canadian citizens live in residential communities for older adults. While fewer older adults in countries within the European Union, New Zealand, and Australia live in such facilities, numbers are increasing (Dupuis et al. 2012; Grant, 2006).

Older adults tend to 'migrate' to residential care communities to improve lifestyle shortly after retirement; to live closer to family members; or, when there is a realisation that extra care is needed (Litwak and Longino, 1987). Giving up a previous home in exchange for security associated with closer proximity to resources, including medical staff (Groger and Kinney, 2007) is important to those who simply no cannot 'keep up'. Even though the move to an RCC may be viewed as 'downsizing', those who live independently within a cottage or apartment-style home often remain autonomous in the ability to own a vehicle, prepare meals and venture away from the facility on their own (Jenkins et al., 2002). Some residents, however, require support for activities of daily living. Continuing Care Retirement Communities (CCRCs) are a unique form of RCCs that offer a relatively flexible continuum of care to meet residents' different levels of functional and social needs. CCRCs typically provide a continuum of living conditions and support from independent living, to assisted living, to skilled nursing or memory care. Many older adults who are well into their 80s, move to a CCRC to 'age in place' as they plan for future needs of support and assistance (Krout et al., 2002). There is great variability in the amount and type of services offered at residential care communities. Facility-sponsored activities are an important component of daily life. Activities provide residents with a social outlet as well as physical and cognitive stimulation. There appear to be, however, both individual and situational factors influencing the likelihood of residents to engage in physical activity. It is well-documented that multiple losses accompany relocation to an RCC from one's home. Stress from relocation can result in undue fatigue, reduced mobility confidence, anxiety and/or depression that can create a feeling of incoherence with oneself and one's surroundings (Bekhet et al., 2009). The ecological theory of aging states that older adults must match individual competency with environmental demands to promote well-being (Nahemow et al., 1973). It is important for individuals to find a balance between personal competency and environmental press, called adaptation level. When communities provide an enhanced environment, it is more likely that residents will successfully adapt to relocation and experience the 'unexpected gains' of integration into their new community (Rossen and Knafl, 2007).

Regular physical activity has been shown to help manage chronic disease, to reduce and reverse declines in functional ability, to positively influence mood and cognition and to add meaning to life in the later years (Heikkinen, 2006; Rikli, 2005; Takkinen et al., 2001). Impaired sight and hearing, pain and/or poor balance have, however, been cited as factors that keep those in care settings from being physically active (Phillips and Flesner, 2013). The relatively new industry standard for RCCs is to offer fitness programming (McHugh and Larson-Keagy, 2005). Thus, many more recently constructed facilities have a fitness centre or gym appointed with sometimes fancy, and often daunting, equipment intended to provide those in ill-health a means to resist ageing and/or reduce healthcare utilisation (Gilleard and Higgs, 2000). A known industry fact is that marketing representatives for RCCs may indeed entice adult children, with loved ones in tow, to sign up for occupancy because exercise is 'good for you'. Upon closer look, these fitness facilities are most often grossly underutilised.

Fitness facilities in retirement communities may be underutilised by residents because many people over 80 years of age have had very little, if any, previous experience of going to a gym and using strength and cardiovascular equipment, or they may associate equipment with the pain experienced in post-surgical rehabilitative services. When it comes to feeling comfortable in a gym environment and/

or anticipating positive outcomes from using exercise equipment, many older adults say, 'That's not for me...my heart couldn't take it' (Cousins, 2000: 282). Furthermore, many RCCs expect residents to take-up exercise on a regular basis at this time in their lives without trained staff to teach and support them (Benjamin et al., 2009). It should come as no surprise then, that planning, implementing and evaluating physical activity programming in residential care facilities can be challenging, even problematic. Most older adults who live into their upper 80s, 90s and even 100s and relocate to RCCs have one or more chronic diseases and experience many interruptions to their health and daily routine. Some residents (and staff) view the RCC as indeed the last station, thinking that it is too late to do anything about their health and well-being (Gamliel, 2000), Still, many older adults have hopes and fears that fuel a desire to engage in activities to help them feel and function better, physically, mentally, socially and/or emotionally. While they have downsized their living spaces and relinquished valued possessions in relocating to an RCC, there is certainly a percentage interested in 'upsizing' their lives by staying engaged in activities that have value and meaning for them (Carroll and Qualls, 2014).

The Palisades at Broadmoor Park continuing care retirement community

So, how can and do older adults residing in RCCs engage in physical activity as leisure?

The aim of the remainder of this chapter is to explicate how an enhanced environment and comprehensive physical activity offerings were co-created by residents, facility staff and university partners at the Palisades at Broadmoor Park Retirement Community. The Palisades at Broadmoor Park is located in the Rocky Mountain region of the United States. It is a privately owned CCRC that offers three living options: independent living, assisted living and memory care. In this setting, resistance to physical activity programming as solely beneficial to a for-profit facility's bottom-line was mitigated by having staff, university partners and residents embrace a person-centreed care and support (PCCS) philosophy that considers each person's needs and respects each person's value, autonomy, goals and preferences (Silva-Smith et al, 2011).

A Wellness Center that included a salon (hair care, massage and manicure/pedicure), a health clinic and a state-of-the-art gym served as a hub for various activities that would draw residents into comfortable, regular contact with one another and support staff. Programming included Wellness Checks, evidence-based assessments of health status, fitness, function, cognition and psychosocial well-being, which were administered upon move-in and yearly after free of charge to all residents (Silva-Smith et al, 2011). The results of these assessments, delivered by university experts in their respective disciplines, were shared with residents and used to co-create multimodal goals that appropriately targeted engagement in community life as well as improvements and/or maintenance of resident functional capacities as desired (Hatch and Lusardi, 2010).

Based on needs and interests, residents had a menu of activity offerings to choose from. A 'Let's Get Started' beginner-level group exercise class, where participants used body weight, dumbbells and bands for resistance training and a more advanced 'Group X' (exercise) class, where participants stood and moved to music most of the class period, were offered twice a week. Tai Chi, Yoga and Aqua Moves were also offered twice a week, on non-consecutive days. A Balance and Mobility class was offered once a week. A focus on fall prevention undergirded all activity offerings. Open gym sessions were scheduled for several hours two afternoons for independent-living and two afternoons for assisted-living residents. The gym was equipped with sophisticated exercise equipment by Technogym™, equipment that provided opportunities to engage in heart-healthy and muscle-healthy activities. An accompanying software system supported by Wellness Keys (USBs) was used to design programmes and track results. Many other opportunities to engage in leisure activities that required physical strength and/or stamina were designed and implemented with and for residents. For example, safe walking routes were identified (and measured) around the facility, inside and out. Raised beds were built to enable those interested in gardening to do so. Community activities, including attending classes at a lifelong learning institute, going to the theatre, to holiday parades, church services and other community events, as well as lectures and sporting events – were abundant. These engagement opportunities were intentionally conceived-of and supported to create an enhanced environment for residents and staff, one intended to change the culture of residential care, one that was viable with staff support from the university as partner.

This author, faculty colleagues and students were engaged in service provision and research at the Palisades for four years. During this time, we were embedded in all phases of community life. As such, we learned how changing attitudes about late life physical activity and increasing support for physical activity as leisure can improve resident (and staff) quality of life and life satisfaction. The following narratives serve as examples of programming designed to help residents maintain functional capabilities, independence and dignity and to foster relation-building, thus thwarting the social isolation that often plagues people living in residential care (Simone and Hass, 2013). Hearing what mattered to residents is intended to engage readers in an important new and transferrable discourse about late life physical activity in residential care settings. The first story is about a class offered to Independent-Living residents; the second is about programming offered to Assisted-Living residents. NOTE: Resident quotes are in italics.

Let's keep moving at The Palisades

If you were to peek into the independent living wing's basement activity room during the morning hours, you might be greeted by the sight of eight to ten women gliding across the room – one, two, three; one, two, three. As they waltz along, postures erect, heads up, arms sweeping side to side, the music and lyrics to *Singin' in the Rain* are inspiring them 'to be happy again'. Shortly after the Palisades opened, Barbara Willis, a 73-year-old dance-movement specialist who had Parkinson's disease, was invited to teach Let's Keep Moving, a class she specially designed 'for those who were feeling the weight of years' as Barbara said, and Barbara was. It is well-founded that dance and dance-movement therapy can provide older adults with a physical activity option that can improve physical function and quality of life, and there are many types of dance that bestow these benefits (Keogh et al., 2009). What Barbara's approach included though, was the purposeful use of activities that helped participants maintain connection to themselves and to everyday life. While she used dance and movement routines to stimulate increased range of motion, balance and coordination, her techniques were not prescriptive. Rather, she met participants where *they* were, encouraging them to 'give me a move, any move' using a technique called signature movements. This technique, otherwise known as instant choreography, encourages participants to connect with *their* movement preferences and needs and to one another. For example, on one occasion, a participant who struggled to hear Barbara's invitation to move in whatever way suited her incidentally brushed her hair aside. Barbara immediately affirmed this small movement expression as 'Perfect! That is just what I needed!' Mirroring the movement back, Barbara engaged participants in the final step of signature movements where everyone remembers and replicates each other's movement, creating a group movement flow. This activity helped participants become *more visible* to themselves and one another and resulted in more movement and more conversation.

Participants in Let's Keep Moving, individuals who had recently given up their homes, friends, and many worldly possessions to relocate to the Palisades, reported via individual interviews and focus groups that this class *helped* them (Kluge et al., 2011). They were (their own words in italics) *moving better and feeling better, realizing a new and improved self, and feeling a sense of belonging*. Most of these women *thought* (their) *dancing days were over*, yet they learned from someone *with a serious illness* that this was not true. This class was *fun*; it was *helping* them to *open up and* to *think of this place* (the Palisades) *as home*. The overall goal of dance movement therapy is to increase a person's capacity to experience the body as a source of information, to affect regulation and to mediate interpersonal relationships (Boyle, 1994), all of which were accomplished. Dance enables participants to 'look beyond' contradictions of older bodies and the values of 'ableism', a system of beliefs that people who are not able-bodied are disqualified from being considered whole and deserving of full social acceptance (Goodwin et al., 2004).

'The Fit 'n Fabulous Palisades Champions'

In the early afternoon, if you were to venture upstairs toward the facility's Wellness Center, you would be greeted with another pleasant surprise: 8–10 residents emerging from the assisted living wing, clattering and clanging walkers and canes, spilling into the 'gym' (as they affectionately called it). During what is usually after-lunch nap-time, the women progressed toward the fitness centre like a metaphorical brass band, moving with intention and confidence, jostling and joking with each other and the student instructors who are there at the door to greet them. The band even had a name; they call themselves 'The Fit 'n Fabulous Palisades Champions'.

The Fit 'n Fabulous programme at the Palisades was developed by the Senior Fitness Specialist at the facility, an experienced exercise instructor for older adults and recent graduate from the University partner's Health Promotion Master's degree program. The aim of the Fit 'n Fabulous programme was to provide assisted living residents an opportunity to improve strength and stamina. Assisted living residents typically have low fitness levels, cognitive decline and various mobility restrictions that often warrant use of assisted devices. These individuals were no different. In addition, as are many people who move into RCCs, these individuals, as evidenced by the results of their Wellness Checks, were unfit or unused to exercise of any sort. It may have been 20–30 years since they had engaged in physical activity, and they were, even more so than those who moved into independent living, physically, mentally and emotionally exhausted from the stress of the move. Therefore, before being invited to the gym, the Senior Fitness Specialist invited the residents participate in a group exercise class for 3 to 6 months where they learned how to use elastic bands and dumbbells and do balance and mobility exercises. This introductory period enabled residents to gain strength, stamina and confidence and to develop trust, rapport and familiarity with one another and the instructor. Using ongoing physical assessments that were part of the facility's comprehensive wellness programme, the Senior Fitness Specialist determined when participants were ready to use the gym's exercise machines.

Ultimately, 15 assisted living residents were eligible and accepted invitations to attend Open Gym, held 2 afternoons per week. At first, participants experienced some trepidation about using the exercise machines. They were big and bulky and *daunting* (participants' words in italics). Over time, however, with support from facility staff and the University students, gym attendees prioritised gym time, improved lower body strength and developed pride and ownership in the programme (Kluge et al., 2014). They formed friendships with each other, staff and university partners (students and faculty), relationships that helped them maintain regular attendance for more than a year despite the health interruptions common in this cohort. Via individual interviews and focus groups, the Fit 'n Fabulous Palisades Champions told us about their experience:

I really like working out. It's good for me and it is fun! I like the personal attention. (Vera A.)

My body feels better. I'm sleeping longer. (Anita H.)

Coming to the gym has helped my shoulder and my knee. I can't feel anything (pain) *anymore.* (Annette B.)

I am more comfortable on the machines now. I can do it! I feel invigorated after the leg press! (Katie T.)

I like this. It makes me feel strong. I just hope this machine doesn't make my chest bigger! (Janet S.)

When you come to the gym, you get your exercise and social time. (Annette B.)

I definitely feel the camaraderie of the group. It's my livelihood. It helps me to keep going. (Marge P.)

Being active in the gym translated into being active, visible members of the community at large and, similar to the findings of Borglin et al.

(2005), appeared to provide an anchorage to life. In the face of what may discourage most – severe mobility restrictions, diminished cognition and frequent fluctuations in health status among other challenges, these women exhibited a sense of coherence (as busy women) and a sense of control in an environment that may have otherwise symbolised loss of control.

Discussion

This accounting of two physical activity programmes held at the Palisades provides an alternative narrative from the more customary long-term care narrative of dysfunction and decline. The culture created was purposeful (Silva-Smith et al, 2011) and compatible with Hill's (2010) positive aging paradigm that acknowledges late life loss as inevitable but asserts that resources can be recruited not so much to mitigate age-related decline, but to maximise purpose in life and life satisfaction. Key conceptual components of the physical activity programmes were based on a commitment to engage residents in conversations about their perceived needs and interests in integrating physical activity into their daily lives.

Relocation to a residential care facility can be difficult. Changing physical and psychological health that warrants a move from independent to supported living tends to put older adults at risk for diminishing life satisfaction, morale and well-being (Hvalvik and Reierson, 2011). A thoughtfully designed facility and living experiences co-created by facility staff, university partners *and* the Palisades residents encouraged engagement in physical activity that resulted in physical and psychological benefits and social engagement. Activity time during the day increased. Lower body strength and stamina improved, and a sense of feeling *fitter* and *better* prevailed. As important, residents developed new friendships that helped them find acceptance and create a sense of belonging in their new place of residence.

While there has been no agreement on what constitutes the 'rather amorphous, multilayered, and complex' concept of quality of life (Walker and Mollenkopf, 2007: 4), residents told us that the culture we created helped foster an improved sense of well-being and life satisfaction. Hill's (2010) notion that the old-old have latent potential was realised by many of the Palisades residents who engaged in physical activity programming. There were multiple benefits and gains that appeared to promote integration and enhance quality of life in multiple dimensions. Participants found meaning and feelings of security when engaging in physical activity programming. They 'upsized' their lives by *getting out* of their apartments to the activity rooms and/or gym *on a consistent basis, testing their limits, having fun, and doing new things – more than* (they) *ever imagined.* The fact that this programme was facilitated by university faculty who were up-to-date on appropriate assessment protocol and that safe, effective physical activity programming was delivered by an experienced senior fitness instructor and student interns under her supervision is not to be underestimated. It is essential to have trained personnel who are equipped to design safe and effective exercise programmes for older adults. It is also equally important for those engaged in supporting older adults who want to be physically active to work in partnership *with* participants to provide experiences that have value and meaning to them.

Looking Ahead

Unfortunately, we are no longer at the Palisades at Broadmoor Park Senior Residence. Despite compelling outcomes that resulted in a positive shift in the industry standard for well-being at CCRCs, after 2 years in development and 4 years in operation, the facility was sold to a company that has not maintained the comprehensive programme we created. Unfortunately, many companies who own and manage RCCs still operate using the industry standard medical model, an often reactive model that addresses health concerns and emergencies after they manifest, providing little investment in promoting residents' quality of life. In these settings, there is usually a one-size-fits-all approach to care services and the underlying ageist notion that those over 80 years of age who are the majority cohort inhabiting RCCs are at the end of the road, all used up and/or not invested in engaging in activities to help them stay as independent as long as they can. While much work still needs to be done, with case examples of what *could be*, as described above, a shift appears to be occurring in favour of providing more humanistic, person-centreed care and services in residential care communities (Dupuis et al. 2012; Hvalvik and Reierson, 2011; Rantz et al, 2008). This culture shift includes an expectation that RCCs will provide physical activity programming that embraces engagement in active living, not only to preserve life, but to enhance it.

How can we change the discourse about older age from fear to possibility? How can we help support builders and managers of care facilities to see older adult residents as wanting to be active – to engage – in order to thwart sedentariness and depression and increase confidence and joy?

Hopefully, this chapter has provided some insight about how we might 'play' in the residential care playground. I assure you that many people residing in these communities hope to make a life for themselves, with your support, which is as rich a life as possible. They desperately want those 'in charge' to see them as the people they are as well as who they still may be able *to become*.

References

Bekhet AK, Zauszniewski J and Nakhla W (2009) Reasons for relocation to retirement communities: a qualitative study. *Western Journal of Nursing Research* 31(4): 462–79.
Benjamin K, Edwards N and Caswell W (2009) Factors influencing the physical activity of older adults in long-term care: administrators' perspectives. *Journal of Aging and Physical Activity* 17(2): 181–195.
Borglin G, Edberg AK and Hallberg IR (2005) The experience of quality of life among older people. *Journal of Aging Studies* 19(2): 201–220.
Boyle DE (1994) The use of dance/movement therapy in psychosocial nursing. In: PL Chinn and J Watson (eds) *Art and Aesthetics in Nursing*. New York: National League for Nursing Press, pp. 301–316.
Carroll J and Qualls S (2014) Moving into senior housing: adapting the old, embracing the new. *Generations* 36(1): 42–47.
Cousins S O'B (2000) 'My heart couldn't take it' older women's beliefs about exercise benefits and risks. *The Journals of Gerontology Series B: Psychological Sciences and Social Sciences* 55(5): 283–294.
Dupuis SL, Whyte C and Carson J (2012) Leisure in longterm care settings. In: HJ Gibson and JF Singleton (eds) *Leisure and Aging: Theory and Practice*. Champaign, IL: Human Kinetics, pp. 217–237.
Gamliel T (2000) The lobby as an arena in the confrontation between acceptance and denial of old age. *Journal of Aging Studies* 14(3): 251–271.
Gilleard C and Higgs P (2000) *Cultures of Ageing: Self, Citizen, and the Body*. Harlow, UK: Pearson Education Limited.
Goodwin DL, Krohn J and Kuhnle A (2004) Beyond the wheelchair: the experience of dance. *Adapted Physical Activity Quarterly* 21: 229–247.
Grant B (2006) Retirement villages: an alternative form of housing on an ageing landscape. *Social Policy Journal of New Zealand* 27: 100–113.
Groger L and Kinney J (2007) CCRC here we come! Reasons for moving to a continuing care retirement community. *Journal of Housing for the Elderly* 20(4): 79–10.
Hatch J and Lusardi MM (2010) Impact of participation in a wellness program on functional status and falls among aging adults in an assisted living setting. *Journal of Geriatric Physical Therapy* 33: 71–77.
Heikkinen E (2006) Disability and physical activity in late life: research models and approaches. *European Review of Aging and Physical Activity* 3: 3–9.
Hill RD (2010) A positive aging framework for guiding geropsychology interventions. *Behavior Therapy* 42(1): 66–77.
Hvalvik S and Reierson IA (2011) Transition from self-supported to supported living: older people's experiences. *International Journal of Qualitative Studies on Health and Well-Being* 6(4): 7914 y

Iwarsson S, Wahl HW, Nygren C, Oswald F, Sixsmith A, Sixsmith J, et al. (2007). Importance of the home environment for healthy aging: conceptual and methodological background of the European ENABLEAGE Project. *The Gerontologist* 47(1): 78–84.

Jenkins KR, Pienta AM and Horgas AL (2002). Activity and health-related quality of life in continuing care retirement communities. *Research on Aging* 24(1): 124–149.

Keogh J, Kilding A, Pidgeon P, Ashey L and Gillis D (2009) Physical benefits of dancing for healthy older adults: a review. *Journal of Aging and Physical Activity* 17: 479–500.

Kluge MA, LeCompte M and Ramel L (2014). Fit and Fabulous: Mixed methods research on processes, perceptions, and outcomes of a year-long gym program with assisted living residents. *Journal of Physical Activity* 22(2): 212–225.

Kluge MA, Tang A, Glick L, LeCompte M and Willis B (2011) Let's Keep Moving: a dance movement class for older women recently relocated to a continuing care retirement community (CRCC). *Arts and Health* 4(1): 4–15.

Krout JA, Moen P, Holmes HH, Oggins J and Bowen N.(2002) Reasons for relocation to a continuing care retirement community. *Journal of Applied Gerontology* 21(2): 236–256.

Litwak E and Longino CF Jr. (1987) Migration patterns among the elderly: a developmental perspective. *Gerontologist* 27(3): 266–272.

McHugh KE and Larson-Keagy EM (2005). These white walls: the dialectic of retirement communities. *Journal of Aging Studies* 19: 241–256.

Nahemow L, Lawton MP and Center PG (1973). Toward an ecological theory of aging and adaptation. *Environmental Design Research: Selected Papers* 1: 24–32.

Phillips LJ and Flesner M (2013) Perspectives and experiences related to physical activity of elders in long-term-care settings. *Journal of Aging and Physical Activity* 21: 33–50.

Rantz MJ, Porter RT, Cheshier D et al. (2008) TigerPlace: a state-academic-private project to revolutionize traditional long-term care. *Journal of Housing for the Elderly* 22(1): 66–85.

Rikli R (2005) Movement and mobility influence on successful aging: addressing the issue of low physical activity. *Quest* 57: 46–66.

Rossen EK and Knafl KA (2007) Women's well-being after relocation to independent living communities. *Western Journal of Nursing Research* 29(2): 183–199.

Silva-Smith AL, Feliciano L, Kluge MA et al. (2011). The Palisades: an interdisciplinary wellness model in senior housing. *The Gerontologist* 51(3): 406–414.

Simone PM and Haas AL (2013) Frailty, leisure activity and functional status in older adults: relationship with subjective well-being. *Clinical Gerontologist* 36:275–293.

Takkinen S, Suutama T and Ruoppila I (2001) More meaning by exercising? physical activity as a predictor of a sense of meaning in like and of self-rated health and functioning in old age. *Journal of Aging and Physical Activity* 9: 128–141.

9
Physical Activity and Dementia: Tai Chi as Narrative Care

Gary Kenyon

Introduction

Tai Chi is a form of physical activity. The most common image or stereotype of Tai Chi is that it is practiced by older adults, in a park, usually early in the morning. Improved balance and fall prevention are increasingly recognised as effective outcomes of Tai Chi practice. However, this chapter expands the use of Tai Chi to consider it as a form of narrative care with dementia survivors. As Phoenix (2011: 112) points out: 'If meaning-making is inseparable from storytelling, and if storytelling is always connected to the body, making sense of the physical changes brought about by the ageing process calls for new and different stories to be told'. The present discussion will proceed in three steps. First, I will consider the background to narrative care and how it relates to narrative gerontology. Then I will discuss the art of Tai Chi as it applies in this context. Finally I will consider the specifics of Tai Chi as narrative care with dementia survivors. The traditional and dominant medical model views physical activity from a competence and performance perspective and thereby often has very limited expectations from this group. In contrast, Tai Chi as narrative care makes explicit the assumption that dementia survivors are persons with a story, moreover, a story that is still open to new meaning. This second approach has significant implications in the context of physical activity in later life. These two perspectives are not diametrically opposed; however, the first can be seen as an example of a thin story of care and the second, a thicker story of care in that it accommodates the narrative dimension of human life (Bohlmeijer et al, 2011). I have been teaching Tai Chi for 25 years to adults ranging from 20 of age to my oldest student who recently died at 102. For the past 10 years I have been sharing the art with this special group of participants. As an art form, Tai Chi is particularly suited to a personal interpretation and expression of the movements, in contrast to a set of performance objectives.

Narrative gerontology and narrative care

Narrative gerontology is an approach to the study of ageing that provides a lens to see its storied nature. Narrative gerontologists argue that it is equally crucial to consider biographical ageing as it is to inquire into biological ageing (Kenyon et al., 2011). Narrative gerontology proceeds by way of an exploration of the life as story metaphor (Kenyon and Randall 1997; Randall 2014). From this point of view we not only have stories, but we *are* stories. Ontologically, human beings think, feel and are predisposed to behave on the basis of stories. A person's lifestory, or more accurately lifestories, are personally meaningful and therefore give us insight into the way the world is for each of us. Given this emphasis, narrative gerontology is particularly sensitive to the inside of ageing, in contrast to outer ageing. Ageing as viewed from the outside is often not an inviting story since it involves changes that are in the direction of loss and decline and reduced probability of survival. However, with a focus on inner ageing, to which we gain access by listening to the stories of those who are living the journey themselves (as Plato suggested long ago), we observe lives that are and can be restoried toward acceptance, meaning, narrative openness, and ordinary wisdom. For some, the journey may be towards more life and not less (Kenyon, 2011). The list of phenomena to which narrative gerontologists are applying these insights continues to grow and among others, includes the Holocaust, age identity, frailty, suffering, widowhood, caregiving, the ageing body (Phoenix, 2011) and central to the present discussion, dementia.

Narrative care is a term that refers to the intervention or practice dimension associated with narrative gerontology. Narrative gerontologists consider narrative care as 'core care' in that it is considered to be as important as the provision of food or shelter or medication. Narrative interventions attempt to create a setting in which a non-judgemental, storytelling-storylistening exchange is established. This is called a wisdom-environment, as its purpose is to facilitate the expression of the storyteller's ordinary wisdom stories (Randall and Kenyon, 2001), with the ultimate goal of enhanced quality of life. It is important to note that narrative care usually results in improved quality of life for both the storyteller and the biographical agent or storylistener.

Tai Chi and inner ageing

Tai Chi presents us with an understanding of ageing that is very similar to inner ageing as it is characterised in narrative gerontology. Moreover, Tai Chi can act as an effective intervention in this context, that is, it can assist in facilitating the process of restorying and the emergence of ordinary wisdom. This is in contrast to a focus on outer ageing, which presents many opportunities for narrative foreclosure (Freeman, 2011) and even despair. Narrative foreclosure is the conviction that one's story is over, that there is nothing new to be expected, and there is a sense of just waiting out the end. Older adults are particularly vulnerable to this experience in so far as they internalise cultural metaphors of decline. Frail or dementing older adults are even more at risk, given their gradually improving, but still most common, living environment in long term care settings Nevertheless, narrative foreclosure is a premature conviction since the person is still alive and their story continues.

Tai Chi is, at once, a particular type of physical activity, a martial art and a form of moving meditation. For the most part learning Tai Chi does not involve control or analysis or the accumulation of intellectual knowledge. Important concepts in Tai Chi, following Taoist philosophy, include yielding and adhering, investing in loss, letting go, becoming soft (Kenyon, 2011; Liao, 2007; Mitchell, 1988; Zee, 2002). The journey progresses in Tai Chi, whether viewed as physical activity-martial art, or as moving meditation, as a function of our ability to accept and surrender to what is happening in the present moment. It is important to note that surrender and acceptance does not mean giving-up and passively becoming resigned to the present situation, nor is it equivalent to narrative foreclosure.

The core concepts in Tai Chi are Yin and Yang, which represent female and male energies, respectively. From a Taoist point of view, life itself is said to consist of male, aggressive energy; in other words, human life is a stressor. The hallmark of Tai Chi is the Yin, or female, principle. It is through yielding and accepting that we are able to neutralise the yang energy and bring balance to a situation. As one of my former students once said, Tai Chi helps you to step back and get a larger view. This means that there is a third way to respond to situations beyond fight and flight, both of which are fear and ego based. That is, we fear what has happened in the past and are anxious about what may happen to us in the future. Thus, there is, what some would argue, a hard-wired control response. These conditions do not operate in the present moment.

Tai Chi is about learning to move with changes. Ageing is also about learning to move with change and to let go of expectations. There is nothing easy or simple about this approach. It requires that we are willing to show up to our present situation, whether it is reading our lifestories (Randall and McKim, 2008) or practicing Tai Chi, and to be open, flexible and vulnerable. This journey is also not easy since we all have a multitude of forms of denial and areas of resistance. An emphasis on inner ageing has the potential to result in personal meaning, wisdom and a journey to more life; however, it progresses at its own speed and in even unexpected directions. We can learn that there is strength in diminishment and loss, that becoming smaller can give us access to a larger story where we may find peace and stillness, about which I will say more shortly. It is for these reasons that both Tai Chi and narrative gerontology can be considered as spiritual approaches to ageing, in the broad sense of that term.

Let us now consider Tai Chi and the ageing body. A traditional Tai Chi class consists of warm-ups, which may include Chi Kung movements, which are individual exercises derived from the form, and form practice itself. The primary goal of a Tai Chi session is to *relax*. Learning to perform the movements correctly is a secondary goal of the practice, of course keeping in mind the avoidance of injury. Tai Chi is an art form, not only in the martial sense, but also in the sense that the body, mind and spirit become a personal canvas that is worked on as we change over time. There is no end to the refinement of one's Tai Chi practice at all 3 levels. Moreover, the beauty of Tai Chi is that it can be adapted to almost any situation.

We learn to relax in 3 ways in Tai Chi. First, the atmosphere of the class is gentle, mutually respectful and non-judgemental. Participants experience a feeling of camaraderie and there is no competition. In other words, a wisdom environment is created. Second, class participants need to focus on the particular movement being practiced, and third, it is necessary to gently coordinate one's breathing with the movement. The combination of these elements brings about a slowing of the thinking mind, what in Tai Chi is called the *monkey mind*. To the extent that this is possible, there is an experience of stillness, deep relaxation and peace, along with the physical benefits of the exercise. This is the Chi in Tai Chi. From the perspective of Tai Chi, this chi or stillness is already in us, waiting, so to speak, for us to slow down, return to the present moment, and breathe.

Tai Chi, narrative care and dementia

I have been teaching Tai Chi to frail older adults and dementia survivors for 10 years. The settings for the classes include a hospital-based Veterans' unit, a private retirement residence and two groups in a nursing home. The nursing home classes include one group with physical frailty and early dementia and a group in an Alzheimer unit. The classes are 30 minutes in duration, 1 day a week. All movements are performed from a seated position and are based on a seated Tai Chi programme which I designed.

Tai Chi is an effective form of narrative care, primarily because it co-authors a wisdom environment with the participants in the sessions. It provides a counterstory to the master narrative of incapacity and decline, that is, frail body and frail mind, by which this group is most often characterised. Nevertheless, Tai Chi is a different form of narrative care in that it does not use stories as the direct vehicle of the intervention, in contrast to such approaches as life-review, reminiscence and guided autobiography (Kenyon et al., 2011). Rather, it uses the body as the vehicle to physical, emotional and spiritual wellbeing. However, apart from the movements, the basic guideline of this approach is to attempt to create a relaxed connectedness between me and the participants. They need to feel that they can trust me and that I am not trying to fix them or pity them or judge them. I am just together with them as a fellow human being.

The following example will clarify this insight. In some of my classes, kinesiology students from another local university are invited to attend my classes. They will often go over to the resident and assist them to move an arm or leg; they attempt to get the residents moving. With all due respect to other forms of physical activity, the response from these residents is negative. They become aggravated and clearly would like to be left alone. I call the students aside and inform them gently that they are most welcome to participate in the class, but to please not try to impose this approach to physical activity on the participants in this class by having them perform the movements in a particular way, or even at all.

This is an important feature of Tai Chi as narrative care. I inform the participants (I call them my Tai Chi friends) that there is only one thing to do here, relax. You can follow the movements, you can watch, you can have a nap; the latter always gets a laugh. In this way, different participants will gradually attempt to do all of the foregoing. I would argue that no matter how young or old we are, or how frail or fit we are, we are always trying to measure up, to accomplish something. In the case of older adults there has been a long life of reinforcing this attitude; however, it is equally significant, for example, in the case of younger athletes, who often experience narrative foreclosure (Phoenix, 2011). In

Tai Chi as Narrative Care 97

this way, Tai Chi as narrative care constitutes an alternative approach and a challenge to goal-oriented performance.

Narrative foreclosure occurs due to the fact that the participants feel they have failed or are inadequate. In fact, some class members tell me that it has been a very long time, if ever, that they can just be themselves. Because of this fact, and since new participants periodically join the class, I regularly share the relaxation speech above. I also tell them that this is Tai Chi philosophy and not just a consolation prize. The result is that most of the participants in my classes experience enhanced narrative openness by trying something new. Many also experience peace and stillness, what I call the stillness at the centre of the story. With respect to dementia survivors, one of my colleagues says that Tai Chi bypasses the disease and goes straight to stillness; it is like the disease is not there during the class (Helen Ijsselmuiden personal communication). They can sense that something meaningful and good is happening, something beyond the monkey mind with its emotional turmoil and confusion. Quiet music is another aspect of the class that enhances stillness. In addition, I mention to them that Tai Chi is made up of movement and stillness, so that in between the movements we *do nothing*. In one class I remember a gentleman saying, 'oh, we are really good at doing nothing'.

When I first began teaching in the Alzheimer unit, I questioned the effectiveness of the programme since many participants did not perform most of the movements. However, the staff person pointed out to me that these folks, when not in the Tai Chi class, do not sit still and they are often agitated and anxious. She observed that most stay for the 30 minutes; they are either calm and observing or quietly listening to the music with eyes closed. In this class, when I sense the stillness in the group, I stop talking and just sit with them. The stillness can be palpable! Is it possible that, having lost so much, these participants can be more open to the stillness at the centre of the story? What a gift to the teacher, since the stillness is co-authored by all of us in the group. In fact, this is another aspect of Tai Chi as narrative care. I periodically remind the group that they need to show up or I will not be invited back to teach and that they are as important as I am to the class. This usually brings smiles and nods of recognition. My purpose in making this suggestion is to encourage the participants to feel that they play a meaningful role in the activity, that they are co-authoring this biographical encounter.

There are no expectations concerning performance of the movements, and the classes follow the *Groundhog Day* 'theory'. This insight is based on the film starring Bill Murray, who awakened each day to an unchanged world. In this context, it means that I never assume that anything is remembered from week to week, since that may cause someone anxiety. However, there are many surprises and the magic is in the details of small progress, which is of course huge for the participants. As with the mature bodybuilders that Phoenix (2011: 122) studied, there is a gap between the master narrative of decline and 'what some of those people actually do and are'. Sometimes a class member will simply watch me for weeks and then suddenly a foot moves or an arm is raised. If I notice that many in the group can perform a particular movement, I return to it several times and do not show other movements in the programme. Being responsive to their stories in this way is an example of non-verbal narrative care.

Tai Chi is particularly suited to this group due to the fact that the movements are performed at a very slow speed. Based on my experiences I would agree with the basic gerontology perspective, namely, that we should never make assumptions about the abilities of dementia survivors (or any older adult for that matter). A powerful example of this is a former colleague of mine in the philosophy department at St. Thomas University, Canada. He was both a colleague and one of my Tai Chi friends.

After his diagnosis of Alzheimer's he visited my class several times as a guest speaker. He had the class both laughing and crying. He eventually wrote a book with his partner (Drew and Ferrari, 2005: 73). In his own words, 'at first it was incredible, but hard things take time to be *fully* accepted. Yet once we accept the truth, what is there to hide? We are indeed free'. As the disease progressed he did not any longer attend my regular Tai Chi classes. However, one day he suddenly appeared in my class in the dementia unit. It was a moving reunion, and he continued in that class, with his at times irreverent sense of humor, until shortly before his death. As I discussed earlier, dementia, as is the case with other ageing phenomena, has an inside and an outside. The outside has to do with social roles, functional capacity, chronological time and physical appearance. The inside has to do with personal meaning and ordinary wisdom.

The second way that Tai Chi is narrative care occurs by way of observing where the participants are in their story on any particular day. This is similar to the discussion above about choice of movements, which illustrates the first way that Tai Chi is narrative care, but it is also different. For example, Monty would come to class every week for a couple of years until she died. She did not perform any movements and either watched me or appeared to be asleep. One day I asked the group if they liked the music. She motioned me to come close and whispered, 'don't tell anyone but of all the things they have us do here this is my favourite'. Another day I asked her why her foot was bandaged. She called me over and said that she apologised that she could not do all the exercises as before since she fell off a horse, and could she attend the class anyway. I said just be careful with your leg. Two weeks later, I asked her if she had been riding lately. She answered, 'don't be silly, I don't do that anymore'. This is narrative care in that I was attempting to listen to her story and her reality and not my own.

A second example is a gentleman by the name of Woody, a veteran of the Korean War. At the beginning of each class, we would bow to each other with joined hands and he would say, 'origato' (the Japanese phrase for thank you). He would sometimes say that he was tired because this was the second time that day that he had done the exercises. You never know. After about a year, Woody became increasingly frail and could not follow most of the exercises. He said that he was still doing his best with what he had. I received a big smile from him when I reminded him of how we bow to each other, and we did so!

The third example illustrates the point that Tai Chi as narrative care benefits both the storyteller and storylistener. There is always at least one staff person attending my class. Every so often one of them will say something like the following: 'I feel so relaxed, I am a new person, this has changed the tone of my entire morning'.

Conclusion

Both physical activity and narrative care are integral to health and well-being throughout the lifespan. They are equally integral to dementia survivors. Tai Chi, as with many other forms of narrative care, is creative and often very simple. The challenge is to learn to ask the right questions of dementia survivors so that they do not feel threatened and so that they can feel free to *speak for themselves* (van den Brandt-van Heek, 2011). The basic guideline is to be present to each member of the group in each biographical encounter. This process of presence and storylistening is an art form, and the learning never ends. In the case of frail older adults, this means attempting to move with their changes, which are sometimes rather dynamic in terms of time, in that change can be rapid and unpredictable.

I have also observed that practitioners of Tai Chi, who subsequently become dementia survivors, are able to perform some of the movements and find stillness long into the disease. I would speculate that perhaps Tai Chi acts as a kind of brain fitness, and thereby could be investigated as a preventive measure for dementia. In any case, Tai Chi as narrative care, as an art form, provides frail older adults with an alternative to goal-oriented expectations of performance. This freedom makes it possible for dementia survivors to feel that they can still participate in a meaningful activity and even find peace and stillness. Finally, paraphrasing a remark I once heard by the late pioneering geriatrician Robert Butler, physical activity is the closest thing we have to an elixir of life.

References

Bohlmeijer E, Kenyon G and Randall W (2011) Toward a narrative turn in health care. In: G Kenyon, E Bohlmeijer and W Randall (eds) *Storying Later Life: Issues, Investigations and Interventions in Narrative Gerontology*. New York: Oxford University Press, pp. 366–380.
Drew L and Ferrari L (2005) *Different Minds: Living with Alzheimer Disease*. Fredericton, NB: Goose Lane.
Freeman M (2011) Narrative foreclosure in later life: possibilities and limits. In: G Kenyon, E Bohlmeijer and W Randall (eds) *Storying Later Life: Issues, Investigations, and Interventions in Narrative Gerontology*. New York: Oxford University Press, pp. 3–19.
Kenyon G (2011) On suffering, loss, and the journey to life: Tai Chi as narrative care. In: G Kenyon, E Bohlmeijer and W Randall (eds) *Storying Later Life: Issues, Investigations and Interventions in Narrative Gerontology*. New York: Oxford University Press, pp. 237–251.
Kenyon G, Bohlmeijer E and Randall W (eds) (2011) *Storying Later Life: Issues, Investigations and Interventions in Narrative Gerontology*. New York: Oxford University Press.
Kenyon G and Randall W (1997) *Restorying our Lives: Personal Growth through Autobiographical Reflection*. Westport, CT: Praeger.
Liao W (2007) *The Essence of T'ai Chi*. Boston: Shambala.
Mitchell S (trans)(1988) *Tao te Ching*. New York: Harper Perennial.
Phoenix C (2011) Young bodies, old bodies, and stories of the athletic self. In: G Kenyon, E Bohlmeijer and W Randall (eds) *Storying Later Life: Issues, Investigations and Interventions in Narrative Gerontology*. New York: Oxford University Press, pp. 111–125.
Randall W (2014) *The Stories We Are: An Essay on Self-Creation* (2nd edition). Toronto: University of Toronto Press.
Randall W and McKim E (2008) *Reading Our Lives: The Poetics of Growing Old*. New York: Oxford University Press.
Randall W and Kenyon G (2001) *Ordinary Wisdom: Biographical Aging and the Journey of Life*. Westport, CT: Praeger.
van den Brandt-van Heek M-E (2011) Asking the right questions: enabling persons with dementia to speak for themselves. In: G Kenyon, E Bohlmeijer and W Randall (eds) *Storying Later Life: Issues, Investigations and Interventions in Narrative Gerontology*. New York: Oxford University Press, pp. 338–353.
Zee W (2002) *Wu Style Tai Chi Chuan: Ancient Chinese Way to Health*. Berkeley, CA: North Atlantic Books.

10
The Multidimensionality of Pleasure in Later Life Physical Activity

Cassandra Phoenix and Noreen Orr

Introduction

Deeply embedded within Western society, the prevailing master narrative associated with growing older is the narrative of decline (Gullette, 1997). This narrative depicts ageing as natural and an inevitable downward trajectory of physical deterioration, as 'a tragedy of accumulating deficits, diminishing reserves, and deteriorating attractiveness and strength' (Randall and McKim, 2008: 4). It is oppressive – downplaying the deeper dimension of ageing and presenting ageing as passively getting rather than actively growing old. This has consequences for the meanings and motivations attributed to physical activity in the sense that ageing can be seen as a problem, to which regular physical activity offers a solution.

More recently, Gilleard and Higgs (2013: 20) have discussed a shift in how growing older is experienced and framed, asserting that narratives surrounding the 'new ageing' differ from those which throughout modernity largely emptied the ageing body of any other meaning aside from health and social care. For them, the new ageing body is as much about 'possibility as well as constraint, the site for new practices and new freedoms as much, if not more than, for old vulnerabilities'. As part of this, *doing* activity (physical, social, mental) and *being* what Katz (2000) refers to as a 'busy body', has become a key feature of new, or 'third age' identities. This alternative approach to ageing has, or course, not emerged without criticism. Cautions have been raised regarding the homogenisation, normalisation and subsequent expectation of one's commitment to age 'successfully' (see Pike, this volume) through their will to health and the conflation of 'keeping fit' with keeping old age at bay (see Gilleard and Higgs, this volume), a line of thinking which does little to resist or challenge the ageist undertone that shapes and is framed by the decline narrative (Phoenix and Smith, 2011).

Critically informed research into experiences of later life sport and physical activity can make a valuable contribution to our understanding of this shifting landscape and the debates concerning the physically active ageing body that ensue. For example, previous research in this domain has shown how physically active older adults can nurture nuanced forms of ageing embodiment that may, over time, embrace, negotiate and resist a changing corporeality (e.g. see Tulle, 2007; Phoenix and Sparkes, 2009; Griffin, 2010; Dionigi et al., 2013). This work offers a point of departure from the foreclosing capacity of decline narratives. Furthermore, in some instances at least, it simultaneously interrogates the prescriptive and restrictive directives that can act upon older adults under the guise of 'active' or 'successful ageing'.

In this chapter, we extend this work by reflecting on a topic that has gone somewhat unnoticed when considering the possibilities, constraints, new practices and freedoms that later life involvement in sport and physical activity might provide. That is, the notion of *pleasure*. While acknowledging that pleasure lacks a stable definition, for the purpose of this chapter, we follow Smith's (1980: 75) description of pleasure as being the diverse emotions that make a person 'feel good', including 'happiness, joy, fun, sensuality, amusement, mirth, tranquility'. Massumi's alignment of pleasure with the notion of affect also resonates in the sense that experiences of pleasure involve "nothing less than the perception of one's own vitality, one's sense of aliveness, of changeability (often described as 'freedom')" (cited in Thrift, 2008: 180).

We begin our chapter by noting the curious absence of pleasure within a number of relevant literatures and offer suggestions as to why this might be the case. We then highlight the importance of pleasure before briefly signposting where and how pleasure has been dealt with in ways that could have some synergies with our understanding of the 'new ageing'. At this point, our focus shifts onto our own empirically informed attempts to construct a typology of pleasure for physical activity in older age. We conclude the chapter with a discussion of selected theoretical, methodological and practical implications of pursuing the pleasures of physical activity in older age.

(Absent) pleasures of physicality

Pleasure is an under-researched and under-theorised concept within social and medical sciences (Booth, 2009; Coveney and Bunton, 2003). The reasons for this are numerous and include a preference to study illness rather than factors surrounding health, prejudice in what's considered 'serious' academic pursuit and the perceived frivolity of pleasure in the face of more earnest struggles against alarmist topics such as the *global physical inactivity pandemic* (Das and Horton, 2012), and the uncharted impact of an ageing population. For Booth (2009: 133), this neglect is symptomatic of the condemnation throughout Modernity of physical pleasures that awakened enjoyment, pride and undisciplined impulses to the extent that devotees of physical activity came to justify their practices on the basis of external factors including health preparation for war. Such politics of pleasure, Booth argues, have resulted in a 'prejudice against pleasure in the academy and in state policy'. These continue to be reflected in dominant narratives circulating within the subcultures of sport, fitness and health, which continue to promote instrumental over sensuous kinds of pleasure with performance and health outcomes taking precedent (Smith Maguire, 2008).

Paying analytical attention to pleasure is important because it is integral to understanding how humans interact with each other and their environment in ways that promote health or create disease (Coveney and Bunton, 2003). It is also important because although current health promotion initiatives largely assume that cognitive forces alone govern behaviour, enjoyment and pleasure are central in maintaining people's habitual health behaviours (Jallinoja et al., 2010). A focus on the pleasures experienced in and through an ageing body, similar to that currently emerging in relation to later life sexuality (e.g. Sandberg, 2013), can also offer a different dimension to ageing embodiment that goes beyond the narrative of decline. This might involve, for example, providing a vocabulary with which older adults can make pleasure thinkable alongside an ageing, changing body and the passage of time.

Turning to the small amount of research that *has* involved an interest in pleasure and human movement, the focus has tended to be on high level, sporting endeavors such as bodybuilding (Monaghan, 2001), men's rugby (Pringle, 2009), marathon swimming (Throsby 2013) and fell running (Nettleton 2013; see also Nettleton, this volume). This work has illustrated how the process of intensive training changes how the body *feels* when it is being exerted to the extent that intensive activity can become a pleasure in and of itself. Moreover, as Nettleton (2013) explains, experiences of pleasure are often only understood by those who participate in the activity, who share empathetic understanding of the doing and feeling to the extent that the activity can give rise to a novel form of sociality.

These multiple relations of pleasure can shape bodies, identities and relational interactions over time. But what of the capacity of pleasure to become a lifelong aspiration and accomplishment for bodies as they *move* metaphorically and physically through age and change? Moreover, to what extent might later life physical activity represent one confinement in later life where the *feeling* and *doing* of pleasure might be realised? What does this mean for the pursuit of meaningful ways to 'age well', that deviate from the decline narrative? Our research with a group of physically active older adults goes some way to answering such questions.

The pleasures of physicality in older age

The research used life history interviews, researcher produced photography and a photo elicitation task with 51 physically active older adults (age 60+ years) to understand the role of physical activity in shaping perceptions and experiences of ageing[1]. Our analysis identified 4 different types of pleasure that were experienced as part of a physically active lifestyle. These were sensual pleasure, documented pleasure, the pleasure of habitual action and the pleasure of immersion (see Phoenix and Orr, 2014).

Participants recounted the *sensual pleasures* of feeling the touch of wind in their hair and against their skin when walking outdoors. They described the excitement and satisfaction associated with the sound of a ball or shuttle hitting the sweet spot of a racquet, along with the joy of smelling a freshly mown park. Describing her love of ballroom dancing, Macey (age 77) said 'being in such close contact with my husband when we're dancing is wonderful. I always become very aware of his aftershave and I always like to wear nice perfume'. This notion of sensual pleasure lends support to scholars calling for a move beyond the notion of embodiment and towards a paradigm of emplacement, which takes seriously the sensuous interrelationship between body-mind-environment (Howes, 2005; Pink, 2011).

A number of participants experienced *documented pleasure* by producing written accounts of, for example, walking routes, sailing or trekking adventures (in diary form) and articles for community newsletters. Rose (age 72) explained 'Amongst my greater pleasures is enabling others to enjoy walking in the countryside, from the production of self-guided walk descriptions'. Unlike sensual pleasures, which facilitated feelings of instant gratification and were experienced in the moment of doing the activity, documented pleasure was generally encountered after the activity had taken place. It involved bringing previous exercise occasions into present understandings of the body in time by expanding the experience of being physically active beyond the spaces where it took place (e.g., a swimming pool, a running route, a dance hall).

Experiences of *habitual pleasure* were also evoked by the routines of doing regular physical activity, and the 'agentic field of action' that was enlarged as a result (Shilling, 2008: 13). Habit provided a sense of structure and purpose to everyday life. This seemed especially important during periods of transition such as retirement, relocation or becoming widowed. In this context, routinised behaviour seemed to provide the participants with feelings of control over a new chapter in one's life. Habit ensured that physical activity was accomplished, even on the days when motivation waned. It was this feeling of 'mind over matter' that came to be interpreted as something which was pleasant. Describing the weekly T'ai Chi classes he attends, Dominic (age 78) explained 'Some mornings you wake up and you think "oh, I feel a bit grotty this morning" and I think no, once you've missed it once, the temptation is to say every time I feel a bit grotty that I won't do it, and in fact, I always feel great afterwards. I feel absolutely wonderful afterwards and then I feel happy that I made myself go'.

Although participants may have gained pleasure from this aspect of habitual continuity, Throsby (2013) problematises embodied pleasures that are derived from the domain of challenge and overcoming. For her, it can draw the focus towards sensory deprivation and in some instances, bodily suffering at the expense of embodied pleasures of physicality. The mantra of 'mind over matter', Throsby argues, while useful in initiating and perhaps maintaining certain (habituated) health behaviours, can also dissociate mind from body and reduce the body's capacity to engage with the activity in such a way that it becomes an end in itself, rather than (or as well as) a means to an end.

Immersion enabled participants to consider, escape from and/or gain perspective on issues demanding attention in their everyday life and was another pleasurable aspect of physical activity. For example, describing her Zumba dance class, Josey (age 65) exclaimed 'It makes you feel happy. If you are worried about anything, or if anything is on your mind, you forget about it for an hour and just get sucked in to the music'. Immersion was, therefore, an affectively transformative experience (Throsby, 2013), and participants reported an improved sense of wellbeing as a result. Immersion in one's activity required a focus of body and mind that was often achieved through movement. This allowed the participants to detach themselves from existing pre-occupations. In this sense, like sensual pleasure, pleasure through immersion was at its most heightened 'in the moment' of doing the activity.

The notion of detachment that was embedded within this form of pleasure did not only relate to daily concerns. For some of the older adults, it also referred to people. Immersion provided a route to 'me time' by allowing a sense of identity detached from others (Throsby, 2013). Hill walker Colin (age 69) alluded to this when he described his love of walking in the Scottish Highlands:

> 'I just love it because it's totally committing. You're in the middle of nowhere and you're on your own...I like the feeling that you've got to do it right, you know, the navigation matters, it's a matter of survival really, you've got to do it right. It keeps you incredibly focused. I like that. I like having something I can really focus on'.

In the process of detaching from everyday concerns and people, as Colin's account also illustrates, pleasure through immersion was often achieved by a person's *felt* attachment to place (see Andrews et al., 2014).

Theoretical, methodological and practical implications

Bringing the notion of pleasure to the fore of research into later life physical activity has theoretical, methodological and practical implications. Theoretically, it demonstrates the importance of approaching pleasure as a multidimensional concept. This involves a need to distinguish between different types of pleasure that might be experienced in different spaces and at different times. Indeed, the taking place of pleasure illustrated in this chapter and elaborated upon more fully elsewhere (see Phoenix and Orr, 2014), goes some way to broaden our understanding of how pleasures intersect within assemblages of bodies, objects and spaces. This provides an interesting starting point for discussions around how we might consider the accessibility of pleasures through physical activity, particularly for those older adults who do not experience the sensations of movement itself as something pleasurable. For these individuals, documenting their activity *after* it has taken place, enjoying a warm shower, accomplishing a sense of structure and routine in their lives around an exercise habit might all be avenues where pleasures can be encountered. This line of analysis has the potential to further develop recent theorising around the 'taking place' of health and well-being, whereby 'wellbeing might not be taken *from* the environment but instead might emerge *as* the affective environment' (Andrews et al., 2014: 210).

It also contributes to Nettleton's (this volume) argument for a carnal sociology that attends to the visceral basis of meaning and 'doing usefully' that complements contemporary sociological approaches to physical activity. These, she asserts, may be inclined to privilege health regimens and related notions of governance. Such governance and blame culture is evident in a current masternarrative operating within the domain of physical activity and health, which warns of a *global physical inactivity pandemic* (Lancet, 2012); a 'pandemic' that is situated within current context of demographic change, and in particular, a rising numbers of older (inactive) adults. As a consequence, it works to damage the identity of older adults by positioning them as the least active group in a society where being active is highly valued (see Piggin and Bairner, 2014 for further critique).

For Nelson (2001), masternarratives largely operate beyond awareness, subtly reflecting the expectations that individuals have of life over time. It is this latent quality that gives them much of their power. That said, oppressive masternarratives such as the global physical inactivity pandemic can often be defective in the sense that the normative behaviours that they prescribe can fail to match the individual experiences of group members (Nelson, 2001). In these instances, multiple forms of resistance to dominant, damaging masternarratives are possible and opportunities exist for counterstories to flourish (see Phoenix and Smith, 2011). Counterstories are the stories which people tell and live that offer resistance to dominant metanarratives (Nelson, 2001). It is in the telling and living of counterstories that people can become aware of new possibilities. To that end, the pleasures of physicality in older age have the capacity to enable new possibilities not only in terms of how people might experience their ageing body, but also in the (counter)stories that are told about them.

Resisting identity damaging storylines that emphasise decline and restrict the meaning of physical activity to the management and prevention of ill health and dependency alone is certainly appealing. That said, one must remain equally mindful of the dangers associated with replacing one set of expected normative behaviours with another. By advocating the potential of pleasure to enrich understandings and experiences of physical activity in older age, we are not proposing that pleasure becomes a mandatory outcome of exercise encounters. Nor are we suggesting that physical activity is a pleasurable experience to all people, at all times. Movement patterns can be unfamiliar and laborious, bodies can feel uncomfortable, fitness can allude and bad weather can prevail (e.g. see Ekkekakis, 2010). However, making time and space for the pleasures of physical activity to be realised could initiate experiences even when and where they are least expected.

The methodological implications of this work relate to questions surrounding the suitability of qualitative investigations informed by a linguistic epistemology to examine embodied, affective phenomena (Cromby, 2011). For Cromby, affective phenomena are known corporeally before they are identifiable through narrative. Thus, it follows that participants' descriptions of pleasure (particularly sensory pleasures) are already at once removed from its occurrence (see also Shilling, 2003). Having acknowledged this tension, one might also argue that somewhat ineffable forms of experience must at some point be transformed if we are to make meaning and communicate them in intelligible ways to the other. Frank's (2010) perspective on this ongoing debate follows that although conventional understanding assumes that individuals have experiences and then tell stories that represent those experiences, this temporality can be reversed to put the story before the experience. Drawing from the work of Mattingly (1998), Frank proposes that there is no reality without narrative and that it is because we have stories that we are able to believe we are having experiences. For Frank, experience is, therefore, nothing more than an enactment of pre-given stories. This ongoing debate is likely to become increasingly nuanced as the *affective turn* within the social sciences continues (Clough and Halley, 2007). That noted, we would suggest that just as an exclusive focus on measures of cognition in a numerical form can limit understanding of how pleasures operates in the context of later life physical activity, so too can a preoccupation with talk.

In response to calls for the multi-sensorial experience of physical activity to be taken seriously (e.g. Allen-Collinson, 2009; Sparkes, 2009), our research with older adults incorporated photographic interviews as a means of encouraging participants to 'grasp at' the sensory experiences of the ageing, physically active body (Orr and Phoenix, 2014). This technique illuminated how, when appropriate for the research questions, there is much to be gained by utilising a variety of data collection techniques that go beyond more established forms of data collection such as focus groups, auto-photography and participant observation. For example, participatory sensory ethnography (Stevenson, 2014), autophenomenography (Allen-Collinson, 2012), and geo-narratives (Bell et al., 2015; see Bell and Wheeler, this volume) are all particularly suited to capturing notions of pleasure, feeling, emotion, affect and so forth.

In relation to the implications that this research has for policy, we contend that the physical activity recommendations and guidelines frequently presented for older adults in health policy are often disconnected from the everyday experiences of those that it aims to serve. In our experience of working within this domain for over a decade, older adults are rarely cognisant of prescriptive figures concerning frequency, intensity, time and type of activity. Often, disease prevention does not form the singular or even primary motivation for being physically active. Indeed, many of our 'already active' participants also live with chronic illnesses such as heart disease, Parkinson's disease, chronic obstructive pulmonary disorder, arthritis and cancers. Instead, older adults come to, leave, return to and remain physically active throughout their ageing process for a number of reasons including the status of their relationships with significant others (caring, cared for, supportive, discouraging); their ability to see themselves as, or embrace the identity of, an (older) person who exercises; and the various pleasures that they experience from being physically active across different times and spaces.

Thus, it is perhaps no surprise that '[T]he public health problem of physical inactivity has proven resistant to research efforts aimed at elucidating its causes and interventions designed to alter its course' (Ekkekakis et al., 2011: 641). This has led to researchers such as Das and Horton (2012) to conclude that more of the same kind of research (that is, that demonstrating the health benefits of physical activity and cognitive forces informing behaviour change) is not enough. These authors emphasise that there is a critical need to move away from exclusively relying on advising individuals to become more active and seriously consider how we can change social, cultural and physical environments that enable this to happen. We feel that an awareness of how pleasures operate within the context of later life physical activity is a fruitful step forward this regard. That said, 'more of the same' with regards to how we conceptualise pleasure is not enough either. There is a need to talk about the multiple and diverse forms of pleasure as well as provide health professionals with the knowledge and practical resources that might be required to communicate, also educate and foster the pleasures of physicality in later life in time and place.

Note

1. Moving Stories: Understanding the role of physical activity in shaping people's perceptions and experiences of (self-)ageing. This work was funded by the Economic and Social Research Council (RES-061-30-000551)

References

Allen-Collinson J (2009) Sporting embodiment: sports studies and the (continuing) promise of phenomenology. *Qualitative Research in Sport and Exercise* 1(3): 279-296.

Andrews G, Chen S and Myers S (2014) The 'taking pace' of health and wellbeing: towards non-representational theory. *Social Science and Medicine* 108: 210-223.

Bell SL, Phoenix C, Lovell R and Wheeler B (2015) Using GPS and geo-narratives: a methodological approach for understanding and situating everyday green space encounters. *Area* 47(1): 88-96.

Booth D (2009) Politics and pleasure: the philosophy of physical education revisited. *Quest* 61: 133-153.

Clough, P and Halley J (2007) *The Affective Turn: Theorising the Social*. Durham, NC: Duke University Press.

Coveney J and Bunton R (2003) In pursuit of the study of pleasure: implications for health research practice. *Health* 7(2): 161-179.

Cromby J (2011) Affecting qualitative health psychology. *Health Psychology Review* 5: 79-96.

Das P and Horton R (2012) Rethinking our approach to physical activity. *The Lancet* 380: 189-190.

Dionigi RA, Horton S and Baker J (2013) Negotiations of the ageing process: older adults' stories of sports participation. *Sport, Education and Society* 18:3 370-387.

Ekkekakis P, Parfitt G and Petruzzello SJ (2011) The pleasure and displeasure people feel when they exercise at different intensities: decennial update and progress towards a tripartite rationale for exercise intensity prescription. *Sports Medicine* 41(8): 641-671.

Ekkekakis P (2010) Pleasure and displeasure from the body: perspectives from exercise. *Cognition and Emotion* 17(2): 213-239.

Frank AW (2010) *Letting Stories Breath: A Socio-Narratology*. Chicago, IL: The University of Chicago Press.

Gilleard, C and Higgs P (2013) *Ageing, Corporeality and Embodiment*. London: Anthem Press.

Griffin M (2010) Setting the scene: hailing women into a running identity. *Qualitative Research in Sport Exercise and Health* 2(2): 153-174.

Gullette MM (1997) *Declining to Decline: Cultural Combat and the Politics of Midlife*. Charlottesville, VA: University of Virginia Press.

Howes D (2005) Introduction. In: D Howes (ed) *Empire of the Senses: The Sensory Culture Reader*. Oxford: Berg, pp. 1–7.

Jallinoja P, Pajari P and Absetz P (2010) Negotiating pleasures in health-seeking lifestyles of participants of a health promoting intervention. *Health* 14(2): 115–130.

Katz S (2000) Busy bodies: activity, aging, and the management of everyday life. *Journal of Aging Studies* 14(2): 135–152.

Mattingly C (1998) *Healing Dramas and Clinical Plots: The Narrative Structure of Experience*. Cambridge: Cambridge University Press.

Monaghan LF (2001) Looking good, feeling good: the embodied pleasures of vibrant physicality. *Sociology of Health Illness* 23(3): 330–356.

Nelson HL (2001) *Damaged Identities, Narrative Repair*. New York: Cornell University Press.

Nettleton S (2013) Cementing relations with a sporting field: fell running in the English Lake District and the acquisition of existential capital. *Cultural Sociology* 7(2): 196–210.

Orr N and Phoenix C (2014) Photographing physical activity: using visual methods to 'grasp at' the sensual experiences of the ageing body. *Qualitative Research* Epub ahead of print 24 July 2014.

Phoenix C and Orr N (2014) Pleasure: a forgotten dimension of ageing and physical activity. *Social Science and Medicine* 115: 94–102.

Phoenix C and Smith B (2011) Telling a (good?) counterstory of aging? natural bodybuilding meets the narrative of decline. *Journals of Gerontology Series B: Psychological Science / Social Science* 66(5): 628–639.

Phoenix C and Sparkes AC (2009) Being Fred: big stories, small stories and the accomplishment of a positive ageing identity. *Qualitative Research* 9(2): 83–99.

Piggin J and Bairner A (2014) The global physical inactivity pandemic: an analysis of knowledge production. *Sport, Education and Society* Epub ahead of print 10 February 2014.

Pink S (2011) From embodiment to emplacement: re-thinking competing bodies, senses and spatialities. *Sport Education and Society* 16(3): 343–355.

Pringle R (2009) Defamiliarizing heavy-contact sports: a critical examination of rugby, discipline and pleasure. *Sociology of Sport Journal* 26: 211–234.

Randall WL and McKim AE (2008) *Reading Our Lives: The Poetics of Growing Old*. New York: Oxford University Press,

Sandberg L (2013) Just feeling a naked body close to you: men, sexuality and intimacy in later life. *Sexualities* 16(3/4): 261–282.

Shilling C (2003) *The Body and Social Theory* (2nd edition). London: Sage.

Shilling C (2008) *Changing Bodies: Habit, Crisis and Creativity*. London: Sage.

Smith SLJ (1980) On the biological basis of pleasure: some implications for leisure policy. In: T Goodale and P Witt (eds) *Recreation and Leisure: Issues in an Era of Change*. State College, PA: Venture Publishing, pp. 50–61.

Smith Maguire J (2008) *Fit for Consumption: Sociology and the Business of Fitness*. New York: Routledge.

Sparkes A (2009) Ethnography and the senses: challenges and possibilities. *Qualitative Research in Sport and Exercise* 1(1): 21–35.

Stevenson A (2014) We came here to remember: using participatory sensory ethnography to explore memory as emplaced, embodied practice. *Qualitative Research in Psychology* 11: 335–349.

Thrift N (2008) *Non-Representational Theory: Space, Politics, Affect.* London: Routledge.

Throsby K (2013) 'If I go in like a cranky sea lion, I come out like a smiling dolphin': marathon swimming and the unexpected pleasures of being a body in water. *Feminist Review* 103: 5–22.

Tulle E (2007) Running to run: embodiment, structure and agency amongst veteran elite runners. *Sociology* 41(2): 329–346.

11
The Contingencies of Exercise Science in a Globalising World: Ageing Chinese Canadians and their Play and Pleasure in Exercise

Shannon Jette and Patricia Vertinsky

Introduction

Growing concern over the 'greying' of North America, and in particular the construction of ageing bodies as an imminent threat to already overstressed health care systems, has challenged gerontologists and policy makers who pose physical activity as the 'positive' against which the 'negative' forces of dependency, illness and loneliness in old age may be mitigated (Katz, 2000). In recent years, especially, scientists are trying to identify the correct dose of exercise required to prevent or reverse cognitive decline, as well as the best type and amount to promote independent living in older adults (Peterson et al., 2010; Sofi et al., 2011). Framed this way, physical activity fits nicely within the Western gerontological model of 'successful ageing' that, as Cruikshank (2009) points out, brings business standard measures to a complex human process along with a homogenous perspective that overlooks the very important role that class, race and gender plays in determining how healthy we are in old age.

Guided by the prevailing biomedical model with its dualist mind-body philosophy and an emphasis on the specific needs and vulnerabilities of perceived 'at risk' populations, Western health and exercise prescriptions can leave little room for practices of embodied agency, especially where ageing bodies are concerned (World Health Organization, 2002; Bauman et al., 2012). Experiences of pleasure and a discourse of play seem especially at odds with this cultural model of the body and health maintenance.

But what insights, we asked ourselves, might be offered by turning our attention to traditional Chinese understandings of health and geographies of the body that have been vastly different from Western understandings? Although painting with a broad brush, traditional Chinese medical tradition focuses on the flow of qi^1 (the primordial source of all life, or 'energy' that is neither matter nor spirit) through channels of the body (hence treatment of blockages with acupuncture) and maintenance of mind-body balance. Western medicine focuses on the heart and circulatory system as the ruler of the body and is underpinned by a Cartesian separation of mind and body in which the latter is viewed as a machine comprised of discrete parts, and ill health is the result of the breakdown of one of these parts. Differing ideas around the benefits and risks of exertion arise from these varying body ontologies, leading to a divergence in bodily practices that are conducted in the name of health (e.g., the use of Eastern body practices of Tai Chi (see Kenyon, this volume) to maintain bodily balance, while cardiovascular training to strengthen the heart muscle tends to dominate Western fitness regimes).

It was with these variations in mind that we conducted in-depth interviews with a number of Chinese origin women aged 65 and over who now live in Canada and were actively participating in exercise classes or sporting/fitness activities (see Jette and Vertinsky, 2011). Our aim was to broaden our understanding of repertoires of body practices and self-cultivation across different cultures and their convergence in order to advise upon health care policies and lifestyle prescriptions which often lack sensitivity to social location and cultural nuance – as well as being largely oblivious to power relations that they (re)produce.

In this chapter, we provide an overview of key findings from this previous investigation (published elsewhere)[2] explaining how our female respondents combined Traditional Chinese Medicine (TCM) with Western biomedicine in creative ways, with many viewing (and using) traditional Chinese body practices as an extension of TCM, a technique to help them achieve balance (Jette and Vertinsky, 2011). We then explore in more detail the relevance of the concepts of pleasure and play to our participants' physical activity pursuits. In particular, we are interested in (and wish to further develop) our finding that, rather than adopting neoliberal notions of personal responsibility for health based upon a Western conceived calculus of risk, these older women pointed out that their chosen physical activity practices were often undertaken in pursuit of happiness and life balance, characterising their practice of Tai Chi as 'playing Tai Chi'. We relate this finding to a growing body of literature exploring the importance of the complexities of pleasure and playfulness gained through physical activity (and related healthful practices) (Coveney and Bunton, 2003; Frolich et al., 2013; Phoenix and Orr, 2014; Pronger, 2002; Twietmeyer, 2012) and then explore what an Eastern body ontology might contribute to this understanding. First, however, we provide a brief overview of our theoretical framework that helps us to understand the body as a site of both cultural expression and power relations.

Theoretical framework

Our project was informed by Henning Eichberg's broad concept of body culture, defined as everything that people do with their bodies, including the daily practices of exercise, weight control and so on, as well as the ways that these practices are trained into the body and the lifestyle that is expressed in that display. Marcel Mauss (1935: 97) was among the first to focus upon cultural impact and direct the attention of social scientists to 'techniques of the body': 'the ways in which from society to society [people] know how to use their bodies'. He explains how automatic or seemingly trivial bodily actions such as walking styles, swimming or throwing can express an entire orientation to the world as well as the internalisation and incorporation of culture. Building on the work of Mauss, Pierre Bourdieu (1993: 74) suggests that 'habitus', or 'the history incarnated in bodies, in the form of that system of enduring dispositions' articulated the way that a culture – and the power relations in operation – is written upon and through the body in ways that often appear natural or taken for granted. It comprises, he explains, the unconscious dispositions, taken for granted preferences and attitudes towards the world which are displayed in an individual's natural sense of correct behaviour and social order, taste for cultural goods, views of morality, sense of time and so on. These ideas helped to guide our understanding of some of the bodily dispositions and practices revealed by our participants – for instance, the participants' aversion to practicing rigorous (sweat inducing) activities outdoors at particular times of the day for fear that 'bad winds' might enter the pores and cause blockage to qi, and therefore illness (Jette and Vertinsky, 2011).[3]

Also of relevance to our discussion are Michel Foucault's (2003) well known explorations of biopower and the technologies of the self in which individuals come to internalise disciplinary regimes and harmonise their own behaviour with the goals of the state (see also Rogaski, 2004: 300). Hence, not only must we try to understand what a culture 'knows' about health and exercise, but we also need to be sensitive to the context in which such knowledge has been developed, utilised and translated, since the creation and transformation of prevailing health and healing traditions in China illuminate the crucial role of the body in the construction of China's modern existence.

Susan Brownell (2009), for example, details how 'the body' as understood in the English language, has two common characters in Chinese, *shen* and *ti*, the former implying a lived body that is to be cultivated (along with moral character) and the latter associated with 'physique' and the most common character in the language of modern sport. Over time, she suggests, physical culture practices in China have shifted back and forth from being rooted in the character *shen* (*yangsheng*) to *ti* (*tiyu*), depending on the political and social context. It is the first term, *shen*, that appears in the concept of *yangsheng* or the 'arts of life cultivation' that characterise contemporary health and physical culture practices amongst the elderly in China (Brownell, 2009; Farquhar and Zhang, 2005; Yang, 2006). Farquhar and Zhang (2012) point out that in contemporary modern Beijing, one can see life being cultivated wherever there is some outdoor space. Older retired citizens are walking, jogging, playing Tai chi, qigong, stretching and dancing, mostly in groups, and commonly exchange health advice from friends and popular media about cultivating good spirits (*jingshen*), nutrition, and exercise. They contrast *yangsheng* to *tiyu*, the calisthenics implemented during the Maoist period that was intent on building national strength. Following the end of the Cultural Revolution and the beginning of the era of reform and opening up of China to the world, there was a move away from *tiyu* that was reflected in the 1980s fashion (or reactivation) of *qigong*[4], a loose grouping of exercises based on the cultivation of *qi* (Chen, 2003), as well as growing interest in other *yangsheng* 'life cultivation' practices (Farquhar and Zhang, 2005, 2012). Given the shifting social and political context of bodily practices within China as well as between China and Canada in a postmodern, increasingly multicultural world, we were interested to examine how Chinese women living in Canada understand and experience the pleasures of physical culture.

The topic of pleasure (and the related metaphor of play) has recently come into greater focus in scholarly work in the field of Kinesiology (see Phoenix and Orr, this volume; Booth, 2009; Ekkekakis et al., 2013; Frolich et al., 2012; Pringle, 2010), a trend likely inspired by a growing academic interest in affect. 'Pleasure' brings into focus the (biological) body and downplays the (rational) mind, upsetting the typical privileging of the mind in the mind/body dualism that continues to underpin

Western philosophy (Coveney and Bunton, 2003; Ekkekakis et al., 2013). Some scholars (Beresin, 2013; Pringle, 2010; Wellard, 2012) thus note the potential of emphasising the intrinsic pleasure of movement over the current emphasis on extrinsic motivation (that is, health, morality) that was instilled early in modernity as physical education and sport underwent codification (Booth, 2009). The trend continues today: even as we see a fresh emphasis on play (as a metaphor for pleasure), it is ultimately tied to health and used as a promotion tool in public health (Fusco, 2007; Frolich et al., 2013; Gard and Wright, 2005). Pringle (2010), for instance, argues that while many sport pedagogues are cognisant of the value of the pleasure of movement in physical education, few celebrate the educative value of pleasure alone and instead, dominant justifications for physical activity too often rest on instrumental and developmental goals.

Such concerns are not unwarranted as a current research trend in exercise-affect is a focus on exercise adherence. In their comprehensive summary of exercise-affect research, Ekkekakis et al. (2013: 753) suggest that research in the area of sport psychology is moving beyond cognitive behavioural models (based on the assumption of rational human behaviour) to explore the use of pleasure in exercise motivation. The next step, the authors suggest, will be to determine how 'reason and affect interact to codetermine behavioral decisions'. They call for a research agenda in which researchers explore biological (including genetic) mediators of affective responses. Thus, while seemingly looking to overcome Cartesian mind/body dualisms, the goal to discipline and regulate bodies remains.

The examination of the literature on pleasure, play and physical activity brings to light the persistence of the 'rational' as pleasure and play are co-opted by the realm of health promotion. Agency appears limited. It is with this in mind that we turn to the narratives of our participants. What can we learn from their discussions of health, the body and movement? In what follows, we begin by providing an overview of key findings from our previously published study and then more fully examine what their narratives might teach us about play and pleasure in movement.

Overview of previous research: exercise is more than medicine

In an effort to explore the impact of culture and gendered meanings attached to exercise, we recruited our participants from Greater

Vancouver, a richly multicultural community where people of Chinese descent comprise almost 20% of the total population and almost 50% in some suburban areas (Statistics Canada, 2008). Indeed, Vancouver is now being touted as the most Asian city outside of Asia (Todd, 2014). We focused on older Chinese immigrant women in Vancouver given that they are a group more likely to have been exposed to TCM beliefs around exercise, exertion and health as well as Western biomedical ideas. The inclusion criteria for our interviews were Chinese-origin, aged 65 and over and actively participating in exercise classes or sporting/fitness activities. Our sample was diverse in terms of educational level, socio-economic status, the number of years they had lived in Canada and their place/s of origin. The participants also varied in age (from 66 to 80), although all belonged to a generation who were children or young adults during the Mao years, and if living in China (as was the case with 11 of the 15 women) were exposed to the doctrines and ideologies associated with the Communist state and its aftermath, including narratives about the body and health.

Having conducted in-depth semi-structured interviews with our 15 participants in their preferred language – mostly Cantonese – a thematic analysis of results was conducted so that we could examine the women's discursive constructions and experiences of the body and health (and how they were similar or different). While we soon became aware of the diversity and complexity of the responses, three themes were identified. The first concerned the women's use of medicine: they saw serious illnesses or 'big' problems such as heart attack or broken bones as needing to be treated with Western medicine while most used TCM to treat 'small' problems (lingering problems like a cold or malaise). Thus, they discussed how they tended to combine prescriptions from western biomedicine and TCM in their daily lives, often in a pragmatic way. This elasticity in appropriating a variety of health and body practices has been elaborated by Allchin (1996: S111) who points out how, historically, at least 'the Chinese have been far more concerned about efficacy in practice than about explanation'. More recently, Andrews (2014: 215–216) has shown how, in modern China, Western medicine and Chinese medicine have come to exist side by side, 'like two mirrors facing each other at a short distance...remove one of the mirrors from the scene and the other loses its view of itself'. Just as Western medicine was adopted to meet the needs and concerns of modern China, Chinese medicine has also been modified in its application abroad. Indeed, she concludes, 'there never was and is not now a single Chinese medicine'.

The second commonality pertains to our participants' preferred physical activity practices: a number of them explained that they had returned to (or adopted) Chinese body practices (such as *Luk Tung Kuen* and/or *Tai Chi*) in an attempt to regain health (and bodily balance) following lifestyle stresses that led to what they perceived as health fatigue. Their descriptions of health fatigue were similar to a condition described in the West as 'Chronic Fatigue Syndrome'. There is uncertainty and debate about this condition in the West because there is no accepted test for it, its etiology is unknown, and many medical professionals do not recognise it as a 'true' condition. In contrast, in Chinese medicine it can be explained by two conditions – pathogenic factor and Latent Heat (Maciocia, n.d). Although simplifying the issue, both pathogenic factor and Latent Heat are believed to be linked to an invasion of an external wind into the body that is not cleared properly, disrupting *qi* and weakening the yin/yang balance. The participants thus began Chinese oriented exercise practices to regain bodily balance. While it was deemed good to breathe in fresh air during exercise, it was also understood that one should not play Tai Chi under the trees in the morning because that is where the fog goes and the moisture can enter the body and cause sickness. Fear of sweating generated the same anxiety. One woman indicated that as a child her teachers would warn pupils not to take a cold shower after sweating; pores of the skin opened by sweat could provide dangerous avenues of contagion inside the body.

The final important connection that we discerned in the narratives of our participants related to mind/body balance. That is to say, exercise was seen as a means to achieve happiness or peace of mind that in turn was central to leading a healthy existence. We did not initially ask about the link between bodily health and emotive state (especially happiness), but this connection often arose when we asked the women to list the benefits or 'best thing' about the various physical activities that they engaged in. Regardless of preference (exercising alone or with others), the linking of exercise to improved happiness and in turn to health is a reflection of Eastern understandings of the 'oneness' of mind-body (Lu, 2003). In this view, good health requires a balance of yin and yang (mind and body) and, as Lu (2003: 67) reminds us, the role of TCM and Eastern movement disciplines is to 'circularize, adjust and balance *Yin Qi* and *Yang Qi*'. 'Perhaps the most vivid manifestation of *Qi*', says Lo (2012: 12), is 'its use as a language for cultivating an inner sense of Chinese well-being – a language and technology that has no counterpart elsewhere.'

Expanding our analysis: Western debates about pleasure and physical activity – what does an Eastern body ontology offer?

For our participants, exercise was medicine though not in the biomedical sense; it appeared to be more in line with or akin to other activities (not typically associated with 'health' in the biomedical sense) such as singing, Chinese painting, helping others/volunteering and so on. In this sense, the exercise practices of many of the women were not dissimilar to what Farquhar and Zhang (2005, 2012) refer to as *yangsheng*, practices which may include (but are not limited to) exercise and which are perceived to improve the life of the 'spirit' (*jingshen*). 'Spirit' in this context does not refer to ghosts or one's soul but rather vitality – 'liveliness, positive feelings, intentionality, will, or (good) mood' (Farquhar and Zhang, 2005: 312). In their examination of life-cultivation practices in Beijing that have become a widely recognised feature of Chinese public life, Farquhar and Zhang (2005: 307) found that if they asked people *why* they engaged in these practices one standard answer was 'for health' (*weile jiankang*) or for the well-being of the body (*dui shenti hao*). This response would seem to be self-evident, explain the authors, as health is the goal, and exercise and self-care are the instrumental means of achieving it. However, they go on to make some crucial distinctions between commonsense notions of health and self-care in North America and those seen and heard in China (and, we argue, which also emerged in our conversations with Chinese-Canadians in Vancouver):

> [for] yangsheng enthusiasts...there is no hint of onerous duty. Nor is there much by way of health moralism or an implicit negative judgment of those who do not exercise. Moreover, many practices that have no obvious impact on physical strength of body form also count as *yangsheng* and are explained as good for health. (Farquhar and Zhang, 2005: 307)

Thus, while health is the aim, it appears to be a different view of health – one that requires the integration of mind, body, spirit and one's environment, in large part by focusing on *qi* and the creation of 'breathing spaces' (Chen, 2003). 'Breathing spaces', Chen argues, refer to the 'literal experience of breath work and the production of spaces in all possible senses – phenomenological, social and spatial' (xi). The result, she explains, is that although respiration can be conceived of as a mechanical process, 'breathing practices are considered to be the foundation for spiritual and physical healing' (2003: p. 8).⁵

We wonder, then, might *yangsheng* practices go some way towards answering Cruikshank's (2009: 3) call for a move towards 'comfortable ageing?' Comfortable ageing is preferable to 'successful ageing', she asserts, because:

> it emphasizes ease rather than external measurement, and because we can judge for ourselves whether we are ageing comfortably. While successful ageing implies that failure is possible, comfortable ageing has a more neutral and nonjudgmental opposite. Comfortable ageing also carries a faint hint of emancipatory hedonism, for which we have little time in youth and middle age and too little permission at any age. I would broaden the definition of 'hedonism' to include the pleasures of breathing deeply and being still.

Recognition of the validity of Chinese body ontology allows breathing and stillness to be a perfectly acceptable – and indeed pleasurable – 'health' behaviour. While Twietmeyer (2012) insists that we must learn to take pleasure in physical activity, he reminds us that it may not necessarily be an end in itself. It is culturally contingent and even coincidental, always depending on what virtues and values are nurtured and possessed in particular communities (Phoenix and Orr, 2014). Our study of older Chinese-Canadian women suggests that Eastern understandings of the body and exercise can illuminate pleasures of and attachment to the art of life cultivation that Western health promotion experts might usefully learn from. 'Embodied life is not just flesh and effort; – it is also high spirits and simple pleasures' (Farquhar and Zhang, 2012: 37). Such pleasure offers, perhaps, a surplus, a bonus, an experience of life that cannot be turned to further account.

Notes

1. *Qi*, in its physical manifestation, has been characterised as warm and located in the centre of the body; it is believed that the movement of *qi* (achieved through meditative breathing exercises sometimes in coordination with bodily movement) can transform one's state of mind and health (Chen, 2003). Meditating on the movement of *qi* facilitates the integration of mind, body and spirit within the self and with the environment.
2. For a full explanation of methodology and expanded discussion of empirical findings see: Jette S and Vertinsky P (2011) Exercise is medicine: understanding the exercise beliefs and practices of older Chinese women immigrants in British Columbia, Canada. *Journal of Aging Studies* 25(3), 272–284.

3. We do recommend caution, however, of the danger of defining an Asian body through 'Orientalist' eyes, that is, an artificial creation of a simple East-West dichotomy and corresponding hierarchy of power relations.
4. Gong refers to the skillful movement, work or exercise of *qi* (Chen, 2003).
5. This is not to say that body cultivation practices are apolitical; according to Farquhar and Zheng (2005), they were a backlash against the Maoist era of mass physical culture (*qunzhong tiyu* or body practices oriented towards building the nation through physical education – calisthenics), and in the years of post-Mao reform, explains Chen (2003), 'by breathing deeply and slowly, either with others in unison or in solitary mediation, experiences of public spaces and urban sites could become infused with personal meaning and cosmological order rather than remaining solely official' (p. xi).

References

Allchin D (1996) Points East and West: acupuncture and comparative philosophy of science. *Philosophy of Science* 63: S107–S115.
Andrews B (2014) *The Making of Modern Chinese Medicine, 1850–1960*. Vancouver, BC: University of British Columbia Press.
Bauman AE, Reis RS, Sallis JF, et al. (2012) Correlates of physical activity: why are some people physically active and others not? *The Lancet* 380(9838): 258–271.
Beresin A (2013) *The Art of Play: Recess and the Practice of Invention*. Philadelphia: Temple University Press.
Booth D (2009) Politics and pleasure: the philosophy of physical education revisited. *Quest* 61(2): 133–153.
Bourdieu P (1993) *The Field of Cultural Production*. New York: Columbia University Press.
Brownell S (2009) The global body cannot ignore Asia. In: B Turner and Z Yanhwen (eds) *The Body in Asia*. New York: Berghahn Books, pp. 23–38.
Chen N (2003) *Breathing Spaces: Qigong, Psychiatry, and Healing in China*. New York: Columbia University Press.
Coveney J and Bunton R (2003) In pursuit of the study of pleasure: implications for health research practice. *Health* 7(2): 161–179.
Cruikshank M (2009) *Learning to be Old: Gender, Culture and Aging* (2nd edition). New York: Rowman & Littlefield Publishers, Inc.
Ekkekakis P, Hargreaves E and Parfitt G (2013) Invited guest editorial: envisioning the next fifty years of research on exercise-affect research. *Psychology of Sport and Exercise* 14: 751–758.
Farquhar J and Zhang Q (2005) Biopolitical Beijing: pleasure, sovereignty and self-cultivation in China's capital. *Cultural Anthropology* 20(3): 303–327.
Farquhar J and Zhang Q (2012) *Ten Thousand Things: Nurturing Life in Contemporary Beijing*. New York: Zone Books.
Foucault M (2003) *'Society must be defended': Lectures at the College de France, 1975–1976* M Bertani and A Fontana (eds) and D Macey (trans). New York: Picador.
Frolich K, Alexander S and Fusco C (2013) All work and no play? the nascent discourse on play in health research. *Social Theory and Health* 11(1): 1–18.
Fusco C (2007) 'Healthification' and the promises of urban space: a textual analysis of representations of Place, Activity, Youth (PLAY-ing) in the city. *International Review for the Sociology of Sport* 423(1): 43–63.

Gard M and Wright J (2005) *The Obesity Epidemic*. London: Routledge.
Jette S and Vertinsky P (2011) Exercise is medicine: understanding the exercise beliefs and practices of older Chinese women immigrants in British Columbia, Canada. *Journal of Aging Studies* 25(3): 272–284.
Katz S (2000) Busy bodies: activity, ageing and the management of everyday life. *Journal of Aging Studies* 14(2): 135–152.
Lo V (2012) Introduction. In: V Lo (ed) *Perfect Bodies: Sports, Medicine and Immortality*. London: The British Museum Press. pp. 1–20.
Lu C (2003) An understanding of body-mind relation based on Eastern movement disciplines and its implication in physical education. *Avante* 9: 66–73.
Maciocia G (n.d.). Myalgic encephalomyelitis. Available at: http://www.acupuncture.com/conditions/cfids_me.htm (accessed February 2010).
Mauss M (1935) *Sociology and Psychology: Essays* B Brewster (trans). London: Routledge and Kegan Paul.
McDermott L (2007) A governmental analysis of children 'at risk' in a world of physical inactivity and obesity epidemics. *Sociology of Sport Journal* 24(3): 302–324.
Peterson M, Rhea M, Sen A, et al. (2010) Resistance exercise for muscular strength in older adults: a meta-analysis. *Ageing Research Reviews* 9(3): 226–237.
Phoenix C and Orr N (2014) Pleasure: a forgotten dimension of physical activity in older age. *Social Science and Medicine* 115: 94–102.
Pringle R (2010) Finding pleasure in physical education: a critical examination of the educative value of positive movement affects. *Quest* 62: 119–134.
Pronger B (2002) *Body Fascism: Salvation in the Technology of Physical Fitness*. Toronto: University of Toronto Press.
Rogaski R (2004) *Hygienic Modernity: Meanings of Health and Disease in Treaty Port China*. Berkeley, CA: University of California Press.
Rose N (1996) Governing 'advanced' liberal democracies. In: A Barry, T Osborne and N Rose (eds) *Foucault and Political Reason: Liberalism, Neo-Liberalism and Rationalities of Government*. Chicago: University of Chicago Press. pp. 27–64.
Sofi F et al. (2011) Physical activity and risk of cognitive decline: a meta-analysis of prospective studies. *Journal of Internal Medicine* 269(1): 107–117.
Statistics Canada (2008) Canada's ethnocultural mosaic, 2006 census. Ottawa, Ontario: Minister of Industry. Available at: http://www12.statcan.ca/census-recensement/2006/as-sa/97-562/pdf/97-562-XIE2006001.pdf Accessed: June, 2010.
Todd D (2014) Vancouver is the most Asian City outside Asia. *The Vancouver Sun*. March 28.
Twietmeyer G (2012) The merits and demerits of pleasure in kinesiology. *Quest* 64(3): 177–186.
Wellard I (2012) Body-reflexive pleasures: exploring bodily experiences within the context of sport and physical activity. *Sport, Education and Society* 17(1): 21–33.
World Health Organization (2002). Active Aging Policy Framework Available at: http://www.who.int/ageing/publications/ative/een/index.html (accessed March 2013).
Yang, DX (2006) *Dusk Without Sunset: Actively Aging in Traditional Chinese Medicine*. Doctoral dissertation. Pittsburgh, PA: University of Pittsburgh.

12
Fell Running in Later Life: Irresponsible Intoxication or Existential Capital?

Sarah Nettleton

Introduction

This chapter introduces the unique sport of fell running in the English Lake District and reports on an analysis of the views and experiences of older runners. Informed by a 'carnal sociology', it is argued here that attention to the visceral basis of meaning gives us insights into why people continue to participate in sport in later life. Contrary to contemporary sociological approaches to physical activity which are inclined to presume that older people participate in physical activity in order to comply with public health pronouncements and to act as responsible citizens, the data presented here suggest that there may be other more profound, existential reasons for their sustained participation. Deploying the conceptual tools of 'embodied intoxication' (Shilling and Mellor, 2011) and 'existential capital' (Nettleton, 2013), it is argued that that fell running which is a physically intense activity is transformative and involvement binds participants through a fleshly sociality. This is why men and women continue to run on the fells in later life even when they are cautioned by health professionals to 'slow down' or in the face of normative expectations that they should turn to more age-appropriate activities. Their imperative to run is because they run: an apparent tautology that we unpack throughout this chapter. We begin with a brief comment on sociological perspectives on ageing, fitness and diversity in later life. We then introduce fell running, outline our methodological orientations and introduce the conceptual tools that inform the study. Drawing on insights from the sociology of embodiment, it is suggested here that pre-cognitive practices and the corporeal basis of meaning-making are the reasons why some older people continue to participate in demanding forms of physical activity in later life.

Discourses of ageing and the imperative of fitness

Contemporary social inquiry accepts that growing older should not be conceptualised as a linear set of 'natural' life stages that progress from relative vitality to relative infirmity. Ageing is not 'pathological' but 'normal'. More recently, this 'normal ageing' discourse has been overlain by notions of 'normative ageing', which point to the 'pluralism, diversity and difference' that characterises ageing in late modern society, and 'dis-embeds the normative assumptions of a singular old age' (Jones and Higgs, 2010: 1515). Indeed, it is claimed that there are many ways to age 'successfully' (Franklin and Tate, 2009). Higgs et al. (2009) however, point to the tenacious aspects of this approach noting its affinity with neo-liberal health discourse that induces people to be active. Those born between the 1920s and 1960s have been most exposed to these neo-liberal regimes of governance that sought to inculcate the autonomous healthy self. Moreover, as these authors point out, the 'will to health' is now matched by a further dictate, namely the 'imperative to fitness'. They elegantly argue:

> For older people such notions of fitness lead to exhortations to develop their bodily capacities and behaviours and not give in to 'indolence'. While these may have been beneficial outcomes deriving from a rejection of 'ageist' assumptions about the older person, they also risk labeling individuals as failures within this new somatic culture (Bauman, 1998). Thus, normal ageing even at its current enhanced level becomes problematised and 'fitness' in later life takes on an aggressive and unremitting stance of both expecting the individual to seek out new experience and to display a capacity to engage with the fitness of 'anti-norm'. (Jones and Higgs, 2010: 1518)

Physical activity and the pursuit of fitness are given impetus by health promotion dictats that promulgate 'healthy' practices, which in turn create spaces colonised by commercial interests. Fitness as a site of consumption offers a 'promise of fulfillment' but invariably 'delivers dissatisfaction' (2010:1518). Social scientists recruited to the health promotion endeavour seek to understand the problematic figure of the sedentary older person in the hope that he or she will be amenable to reform (Tulle, this volume). Researchers examine, for instance, narratives of exercising in later life (Paulson, 2005; Tulle, 2008; Phoenix and Grant, 2009) and also identify factors that prevent or facilitate physical activity (Grant, 2001; Dionigi and Flynn, 2007). Conceptual critiques of the 'imperative of fitness' in concert with this growing body of empirical research are invaluable, but here we shift our focus to corporeal aspects of physical activity and argue that there is something intrinsic to the fleshy, visceral materiality of running (Tulle, 2007), and most particularly fell running, that complements these ongoing debates.

What is fell running?

> For more hours than I can remember, a storm has been screaming around me. For more hours than I can remember, I have been running – or trying to run – in the mountains. Now I am lost, utterly. Every muscle in my body is shaking, both feet are blistered raw, every joint aches, and my last reserves of warmth and strength are gushing away like steam.... This I should add is what I do for fun. (Askwith, 2004)

This quotation from Askwith's book, *Feet in the Clouds: A Tale of Fell Running and Obsession*, communicates something of the realities of fell running, a uniquely British sport that has its origins in the northern counties of England. To be sure there are similarities to mountain/ trail running in Europe and beyond; however, fell does retain some distinctive characteristics such as running off paths, a reliance on navigation skills, the scope for runners to select their own route and the need for a familiarity with the topography (for a detailed history see Smith, 1985). The sport became established in the north of England in the 1950s, and today whilst the racing calendar extends beyond the Lake District, this is where many well-known events still take place. A number stand out. The Lake District Mountain Trial (LDMT) inaugurated in 1952 was the first race that took in a series of summits while being run on orienteering lines: the runners choosing their own routes reporting to designated checkpoints during the race. Indeed, part of the challenge is to devise a route that is most suited to the runners' own style, skills, preferred terrain, weather conditions and so on. The challenge too is not to get lost – and in fact getting lost during a race is a common experience. More than any other event the LDMT captures the spirit of the sport (LDMTA, 2002). The 'Bob Graham Round', a circuit of 42 (initially, now more) of the highest peaks in the Lake District, was first completed within 24 hours in 1932. Most of the men and women cited in this chapter have participated in either one of these events and all in many other races besides. Some ran 50 peaks at 50 years of age within 24 hours, 60 at 60 and 70 at 70. Crucially, all have run in the Lake District for decades and continue to do so. Fell running is hard work; it is physically demanding; it can be dangerous. It requires stamina and endurance, but it is also fun. Fell runners can become gripped by the sport, and as Askwith's book title suggests, it can become something of an obsession.

Embodied ethnography: a note on methods and conceptual tools

Despite fell running's relatively minority status, an empirical exploration of these older amateur athletes informed by a carnal sociology (Wacquant, 2005; Crossley, 1995) may well be instructive to debates on physical activity and sport in later life. Carnal sociology encourages embodied ethnography, which presumes the body to be both an 'object' and a 'means' of inquiry. Here the researcher's body comprises:

> a fruitful conduit for gaining an adequate command of the 'culture' at hand, that is, a major *technique of ethnographic investigation and interpretation* in its own right. And one that is especially well-suited to capturing the visceral quality of social life that standard modes of social inquiry typically purge from their accounts. (Wacquant 2005: 465, italics in the original)

Close engagement with embodied practices reveals a shared grammar of capacities and skills which in turn give insight into 'the carnal quality of membership in a group, and thus, the carnal basis of human meaning-making' (Eliasoph, 2005: 169). Data reported here were generated by the author through participant and non-participant observation: attending races, informal conversations with runners and their families, membership of the Fell Running Association (FRA) and attending a FRA course on mountain navigation. In addition, in-depth interviews with 14 men and five women who live in the Lake District were undertaken, all of which were audio-recorded and transcribed. Participants were aged over 55 and the oldest was 83; all were white British and still running. Some were born in the locality, whilst others had moved into the area but had done so many decades ago. Interviews explored issues such as routes into running, the types of races they participated in, good runs and races, less good runs and races, involvement in the organisation of races and times when they had been unable to run, although this last topic was something they seemed reluctant to speak about (Nettleton and Green, 2014).

Although running is a profoundly individual act, it is also profoundly social. The embodied basis of action reflects what Bourdieu (1977) calls habitus which is achieved not through discourse, but 'existential understanding' (Crossley, 1995: 54). However, embodied techniques that are physically and mentally demanding generate more than just 'understanding'; they also foster *existential capital* (Nettleton, 2013), a phenomenological profit which – through its uniqueness paradoxically – establishes solidarity with others who share their passions. Thus *existential capital* is a concept that seeks to mesh embodiment and sociality and implies that carnal practices generate resources that cement social relations. While social groupings invariably harbour difference, divisions and hierarchies, they are also characterised by shared experiences necessary for their collective definition and identity. However the embodied basis of such communality can be overlooked, as is made evident by Wacquant's (2005; 2014) writings on 'carnal connections'. Wacquant suggests that communal assemblage is invariably anchored in the incarnate, and the fleshy basis of sociality can transcend social differences.

The idea of *existential capital* therefore speaks to both Bourdieusian and phenomenological sociologies. Bourdieu's notion of physical capital reveals how bodily attributes are a source of social, cultural and economic benefit. However, modes of capital tend to be understood primarily as markers of distinction with less emphasis on capital resources as a form of collective gain. And, more importantly, Bourdieu's conceptualisation of physical capital relies, I would suggest, rather controversially on a Cartesian body. Drawing on insights from phenomenology, *existential capital* instead implies that there is much to be gained from appreciating the 'lived body'. Leder (1990) for example, urges that we 'form one-body' (p.149) a body not synonymous with the individual, the self or a bounded physical frame but a form that is permeable to, and indeed inseparable from, the wider world. He writes: 'This body's roots reach down into the soil of an organismic vitality where the conscious mind cannot follow', and, he continues, '[t]hrough the lived body I open to the world' (p.173). More concretely, he identifies three modalities whereby 'we realize the one-body relation' (161): *compassion, absorption* and *communion*. *Compassion* literally means to suffer with, 'a process of empathetic identification' which more than merely caring 'about' generates 'an existential shift' (162) whereby bodies share experience 'with';

thus he argues, 'compassion makes one body of us' (161). The one-body modality of *absorption* shifts the emphasis from the moral to the aesthetic and draws attention to the porosity of bodies. For example, in a pleasing landscape, the environment can permeate our senses, muscles, and consciousness. Poignantly, for our analysis of fell running, Leder takes walking in a forest as an illustration of how we absorb the landscape and the landscape absorbs us and thereby collapses the distinction between the material and immateriality of bodies and places. Certain activities facilitate *compassion* and *absorption* and a concomitant sense of involvement – although diverse; he terms those activities that precipitate such association or assemblage as *communion*. These are most readily obvious in religious practices, but what they share is a corporeal basis that is transpersonal whereby the self and the world are inseparable. 'In eating, breathing, perceiving, moving, the body transcends itself through its commerce with the world. Thus each visceral or sensorimotor function can become a channel for the experience of communion' (172). Taken in combination, Bourdieu's concept of capital and phenomenological approaches to the body help us appreciate that existential gains are both individual and social. This is captured in the concept of *existential capital*. This somatic existential gain can be generated in corporeal practices and rituals reminiscent of those explored by Durkheim (1995).

The embodied basis of social solidarity can be traced to Durkheim's (1995) writings on religion, worship and collective consciousness. Working in this Durkheimian tradition Shilling and Mellor (2011) develop the novel concept *embodied intoxication*. This notion implies that activities that can remove individuals from the humdrum of everyday life and involve an element of transcendence can be intoxicating. These practices in turn form the basis of sociality. Durkheim wrote about rituals, totemic worship and so on, but as Shilling and Mellor (2011) explain, this also applies to other 'body techniques' as defined by Mauss (1973). *Embodied intoxication* can be generated by,

> multiple methods and substances associated with the process whereby people are excited, enthused, inebriated, stimulated and made giddy in a manner that encourages them to transcend the egotistic parameters of their bodies. Intoxication is necessarily embodied, though we write about *embodied* intoxication to emphasize that this is a visceral phenomenon that occasions transformations in *experience* as well as consciousness. Conventional usages of 'intoxication' are too confined to consciousness for us to assume the term can be used on its own to signify a corporeal as well as a mindful phenomenon. (2011: 19–20)

Shilling and Mellor's (2011) thesis is that embodied intoxication overcomes egoism most especially when rooted in intensities of embodied pain and pleasure which can occasion corporeal transformation. Such transformative experiences engender and sustain collectivities and find resonance with our data on fell running.

Fell running: pleasures, pains and intoxication

Shilling and Mellor (2014) suggest that sport 'can provide a *potential* route to otherworldly experience, but its transcendent aspects are *contingent*; manifesting themselves when people's engagement in secular sports happens to 'lift them' out of mundane life' (359). Such removal from the mundane is commented on by fell runners as Dave (aged 65–70) comments:

> It's a release from anything that you normally do through the day. You get into places that you're privileged to get onto, you see things that you'd never normally see, and you're with, generally speaking, such a great bunch of like-minded souls, you're getting changed out of the back of a car, you're covered in mud, but it's just good fun.

Not only does Dave reflect on getting away from the 'everyday' but also he makes reference to being with 'like-minded souls' – the absorption in the landscape and the mud. The notion of fun is worthy of further comment in that the pleasure is not straightforward but can involve a heady mix of pleasure and pain. Steve articulates this when reflecting on the fact that not every run or race is straightforwardly enjoyed:

> It happens regularly, you think 'what on earth am I doing out here?' Or if you get lost for one, and you're cold, and you're wet, and you're miserable, you think; 'what on earth is this all about?' I think probably my worst experiences of fell running are where I've been doing mountain trials [LDMTs], because they are long, they are hard, and for me I would be out five hours plus, sometimes six plus, and occasionally seven hours plus, and you're literally crawling on your hands and knees up some mountains, thinking 'what on earth am I doing this for?'

In the oral history data collected and reported in the book *Fifty Years Running: A History of the Mountain Trial* (LDMTA, 2002) one participant recollects with apparent clarity a race he had run over 40 years ago. It gives some insight not only to the ache of the action, but the heightened sensory awareness that running invokes. This is evident in the following account wherein a runner recollects a particular race, highlighting the navigational challenges and impromptu decisions, the aches and pains and the emotion and affect. In this account (as in others below) local place names refer to fells (mountains) such as Heron Crag, dales and valleys such as Eskdale, lakes and tarns, revealing the runners' detailed knowledge of the environment:

> People were going in different directions, intentionally or not, somehow I found my way over the Coniston fells and up Eskdale. This is where I began to feel pain, but pride or something said I must carry on. The legs were hurting but the brain wasn't listening, thoughts of running any distance were quickly dismissed as any rough ground or incline became a reason to walk. After the check point at Heron Crag we had to continue to up the valley, then take a near vertical route over the Scafell range to find something called Round How. By the top, I was on my own, but I managed to locate the checkpoint. I still wonder if Esk Hause would have been a better route. Somewhere after Heron, George decided to retire, or perhaps he preferred a more direct route to the final check at Three Tarns and the bar at the finish. At this point I was incapable of such logic. The rest was just a blur: the calf muscles screaming on the uphill bits, the thighs on the downhill. The Band was agony, at least until the thought of finishing brought a surge of adrenalin, and I managed a jog and a smile to impress those who had finished two hours earlier.

We can hear in this runner's account recollections of pain, fatigue, suffering, incoherence, confusion and pride. This same runner also comments on the magic of the race:

> I like to think of this and a small number of other events as defining moments in my own life. So much gets forgotten but the Mountain Trial will be with me forever. And it's still there now, waiting to cast its spell on a new generation. (LDMT, 2002: 15)

We might explain this in terms of masculinity – the macho performance of men who beat the elements, conquer nature and thrive on competition. However, the embodied gains were appreciated by women too. When talking about completing the Bob Graham Round, Deirdre (aged 65–70) comments that 'unless you're a runner you've no idea'. Running in the fells quite literally transports the participants from their everyday spaces and gives rise to a sense of freedom helped by shedding the paraphernalia of everyday life and can alter one's affective state in ways that are reminiscent of those described as transcendental and spiritual experiences by Mellor and Shilling (2014). As Tina (aged 60–65) puts it: 'I think it is that sense of feeling really at peace when you've had a good run'.

In sum, the data reveal something of the pains and pleasures of fell running and might be understood as examples of what Mellor and Shilling refer to as 'embodied intoxication'. Having had regular 'doses' of intoxication over many decades the runners show little inclination to give up their rituals and habit. The running imperative is ingrained, even in the face of illness, medical advice to slow down and normative cautions to age appropriately.

Running irresponsibly?

The older fell runners who contributed to this study might be considered to be illustrative of the 'imperative to fitness' and the 'normalization of diversity' in later life that Jones and Higgs (2010: 1518) identify as key tropes in contemporary public health discourse. However, while the data reveal that the participants feel an imperative to run, this is not because they are motivated to be responsible citizens or because they feel induced to maintain their healthy bodies. On the contrary, their continued participation in this extreme sport is regarded by some as risky to their health. Albert (age 80–85) laughs when he says: 'The doctor said "you'll do your hips and do your knees no good you want to pack [give] that up"'. Albert' s laughter is significant here because it implies that the GPs' suggestion that he should give up running is ludicrous (see Nettleton and Green 2014). But then the GP was not a fell runner. Yvonne now in her early 60s still regularly trains and finds that:

> people outside of fell running sort of say, aren't you getting a bit old for this, you know, and family sort of said, 'are you sure all of this is good for you', but it's not done any harm so far. Non-runners and non-fell runners do perhaps think you should be slowing down, but people in fell running no.

When asked directly about periods when they hadn't run, most reported that this had rarely happened although it was evident during interviews or informal conversations that there had been periods of enforced abstinence due to major operations for heart conditions, hip replacements, knee operations and so on. Oscar now in his 80s reflected on his 'younger' days when due to illness doctors had advised him not to run:

> In the early 1970s [aged 55+] I had a serious illness and they said I had never to run again, and I ignored it. I used to run quietly without telling anybody... well I was depressed really because I'd run all my life, and so that was why I ran without telling the doctor.

Reflecting on his health troubles which included a heart condition and associated surgery, late onset Type 1 diabetes and various physical injuries, Ed (aged 65–70) was of the view that the 'medics completely don't understand you'. He cited the fact that, 'they fitted a pacemaker, they set it at a minimum rate that your heart will go, and it won't go down to what my resting pulse rate is, which was about 37 to 40 at the time'. Despite these chronic conditions he runs twice a day, four miles by the lake in the morning and a more challenging run most likely taking in some peaks later in the day.

Running in all weathers, in exposed and remote environments, over many hours, when living with medical conditions in later life might be regarded by some as reckless and is out of sync with normative notions of age- appropriate health behaviours. Thus runners' engagement with the fitness imperative does not accord with contemporary neo-liberal discourses of responsible, 'healthy' ageing. Runners are not deterred by health problems or the pains of running and any health guidance is invariably drafted for those who participate in 'moderate' age-appropriate exercise which is something that Ed finds rather irritating:

> I was diabetic at that time, I think it was just bad management I didn't, well I still don't really understand exactly how it works, because if you've too much insulin you end up with low blood sugar and you feel terrible, but you can actually still run, because it's got the glycogen into your system, into your muscles and so on, but you've got low blood sugar so your brain's not working and things like that, but if you have got no insulin in your system at all, you can have high blood sugar and still feel really really bad because you can't convert it, you can't put it into the cells, so you can't run, and it took ages, because there's nothing in the press about how it works, and if you don't understand how it works you can't really manage it. They can say 'don't take it directly before', but if you don't really understand why, and almost all the information you get is for people who

do five mile races, 10K races, things like that, running four hours is a completely different ball game.

Ed, like other runners, had to experiment, often in spite of, rather than with the help of, medical advice. When asked do you ever feel like running less or giving up after such bad experiences he replied:

> No, no, no, no, but it takes your confidence away a little bit. No matter how bad I felt, always when I raced this magical thing happens after about 10 minutes into a race, and your body kicks everything else out the way.

Fell running and existential capital

Fell runners can experience exhaustion along with exhilaration, and this body technique can be understood as a mode of *embodied intoxication* – a visceral, sentient activity that precipitates transcendental affects. The effort, determination and stamina can bring social admiration. In keeping with neo-liberal values which privilege honed, healthy bodies, fell running is an example of socially acceptable, normative intoxication (Shilling and Mellor, 2011). Not only does it result in productive, lithe and disciplined bodies but it also reinforces communality and conviviality. However, as runners age, their participation is presumed to put their bodies 'at risk' from medical complications, illness and injuries. As we have seen, the runners find that their continued running in relatively remote places, in all weathers, for prolonged periods is sometimes queried by relatives, friends and health professionals who are inclined to advise more age-appropriate exertion and suggest that they might slow down and temper their running. By contrast, within the fell running community the imperative to run and to retain fitness is valorised. Those with a fell running habitus spawn *existential capital* through the embodied act of running and become absorbed in the landscape while generating camaraderie with their peers and 'like minded souls'. Embodied intoxication from sustained physical effort and absorption of the landscape means that the existential appreciation of the running is sharpened and serves to affirm the intensity and meaningfulness of the action. This solitary activity engenders strong sociality precisely because 'only other runners can understand'. Although their participation in physical activity in later life may on the face of it appear as though they are complying with the fitness imperative – this exploration of their embodied experiences reveals that their reasons for running are for pleasures which are more profound than merely maintaining a healthy body. Indeed, as we have seen many continue to run when formal medical advice would be to slow down.

Men and women keep on running in later years because they run and have run (Tulle, 2007), not because they are obedient citizens taking responsibility for their own health. The embodied intoxication engenders existential capital that sustains and supports fell running as runners age and provides an important space to resist cautions against running 'irresponsibly'. Fell runners who run in later life do so not because they feel that they 'ought' to, or because it makes them 'healthier' or because of a 'responsibility' for their bodies, but because they cannot give up.

References

Askwith R (2004) *Feet in the Clouds: A Tale of Fell-Running and Obsession*. London: Aurum.
Bourdieu P (1977) *Outline of a Theory of Practice*. Cambridge: Cambridge University Press.
Crossley N (1995) Merleau-Ponty, the elusive body and carnal sociology. *Body and Society* 1(1): 43–63.
Dionigi and O'Flynn (2007) Performance discourses and old age: what does it mean to be an older athlete? *Sociology of Sport Journal* 24(4): 359–377.
Durkheim E (1995) *The Elementary Forms of Religious Life* (1st edition 1912). New York: Free Press.
Eliasoph N (2005) Theorizing from the neck down: why social research must understand bodies acting in real space and time (and why it's so hard to spell out what we learn from this. *Qualitative Sociology* 28(2): 159–169.
Franklin NC and Tate CA (2009) Lifestyle and successful aging: an overview. *American Journal of Lifestyle Medicine* 3(1): 6–11.
Grant B (2001) You are never too old: beliefs about physical activity and playing sport in later life. *Ageing and Society* 21: 777–798
Higgs P, Leontowitsch M, Stevenson F and Jones, IR (2009) Not just old and sick: the 'will to health' in later life. *Ageing and Society* 29(5): 687–707
Jones IR and Higgs P (2010) The normal, the natural and the normative: contested terrains in ageing and old age. *Social Science and Medicine* 71: 1513–1519
LDMTA (2002) *Fifty Years Running: A History of the Mountain Trial*. Lake District Mountain Trial Association.
Leder D (1990) *The Absent Body*. London: University of Chicago Press.
Mauss M (1973) Techniques of the body. *Economy and Society* 2(1): 70–88.
Nettleton S (2013) Cementing relations with a sporting field: fell running in the English Lake District and the acquisition of existential capital. *Cultural Sociology* 7(2): 196–210.
Nettleton S and Green J (2014). Thinking about changing mobility practices: how a social practice approach can help. *Sociology of Health and Illness* 36(2): 239–251.

Paulson S (2005). How various 'cultures of fitness' shape subjective experiences of growing older. *Ageing and Society* 25(2): 229–244.

Phoenix C and Grant B (2009)Expanding the agenda for research on the physically active aging. *Journal of Aging and Physical Activity* 17: 362–379.

Shilling C and Mellor PA (2014) Reconceptualising sport as a sacred phenomenon. *Sociology of Sport Journal* 31: 349–376.

Shilling C and Mellor PA (2011) Retheorising Durkheim on society and religion: embodiment, intoxication and collective life. *Sociological Review* 59(1): 17–41.

Smith B (1985) *Stud Marks on the Summits: A History of Amateur Fell Racing: 1861–1983*. Preston, UK: SKG Publications.

Tulle E (2007) Running to run: embodiment, structure and agency amongst veteran elite runners. *Sociology* 41(2): 329–346.

Tulle E (2008) The ageing body and the ontology of ageing: athletic competence in later life. *Body and Society* 14(3): 1–19.

Wacquant L (2004) *Body and Soul: Notebooks of an Apprentice Boxer*. Oxford: Oxford University Press.

Wacquant L (2005) Carnal connections: on embodiment, apprenticeship and membership. *Qualitative Sociology* 28(4): 445–474.

Wacquant L (2014) Homines in extremis: what fighting scholars teach us about habitus. *Body and Society* 20(2): 3–17.

13
Ageing and Embodied Masculinities in Physical Activity Settings: From Flesh to Theory and Back Again

Andrew C. Sparkes

Ageing, like masculinity, does not mean the same thing to all men. It varies in how it is understood, experienced and lived out in daily practices. This is particularly so when the body is foregrounded in the places where sports and physical activities take place. Here, making sense of age is a gendered process. To illustrate this, I draw upon selected age-autobiographical moments (Gullette, 2003) to explore my experiences of the gym as a particular place in which I simultaneously *do* age-specific gender and gendered-age. My intention is to add to the limited literature on men's experiences as embodied, ageing subjects and to illustrate some of the affective interconnectivities between them. According to Eman (2012) and Shirani (2013), this is an important task because the social processes of gender include ageing, and their interplay generates specific meanings about masculinity and 'growing old' or 'ageing well' that can represent challenges to identity in later life.

In offering this story from the gym, it needs to be recognised that I am not only telling stories *about* my body, but I am telling the story *out of* and *through* my body as a 59 year-old, white, heterosexual, middleclass, ostensibly (able)bodied, impaired male. As Frank (2013) states, the body is simultaneously cause, topic and instrument of whatever story is told. In this sense, the kind of body that one *has* and *is* becomes crucial to the kind of story told. It also needs to be recognised that in telling this story I am producing an edited description and evaluation of myself and others, promoting certain aspects of identity, such as ageing and gender, over others at particular points in it. In this practice of narration, I am visibly doing and performing identity work for the reader who might wish to reflect on their own experiences in relation to mine and how I (we) might tell different stories to construct different versions of body-selves by using alternative kinds of narrative imaginings.

Pectoral pumping and other sensations in the gym

'One more – one more – come on – *squeeze* it out' shouts Lisa to Jaz, a young British Asian man in his mid-twenties as he completes his last set on the bench press.

Waiting my turn, I watch his pectoral muscles jerk into contraction as he exhales loudly, pushing the bar up with shaking arms. Lisa stands close to him, her muscular, defined and tanned body deliberately accentuated by her tight fitting, vivid pink top and black lycra shorts. Her body announces itself as a competitive bodybuilder and professional fitness instructor. Many in the gym secretly envy her body. They aspire to its dimensions, its symmetry and its disciplined, regimented development. Some may lust after her. For others, she is threatening, too big, too muscular, too much 'like a man' and, therefore, a dangerous gender outlaw.

Jaz rolls off the bench. As he stands, I notice the pump in his chest muscles through the thin T-shirt that is wet with sweat.

'Looks like a "push" day', I say to him with a knowing smile that signals my insiderness.

'Too fucking right mate. She's trying to kill me!' he responds looking directly at Lisa.

'If you trained as much as you complained you might get some results', she fires back. Then looking at me with a smile she adds, 'bloody hell, even *he* bench presses more than you'.

I accept my part in the joke. The three of us laugh as I move towards the bench. Before departing to another space where Jaz is to be subjected to more intense chest, shoulder and triceps exercises, Lisa slowly scans the gym. Without warning she exclaims, 'I've just realised, I'm the second oldest person in here'.

We laugh again as I look around the gym at the surrounding, mostly male, 20 something, bodies in action. I quickly realise that my 59 year old own corporeality is the reference point for Lisa's statement. Right now, at 19.30 on a Wednesday evening in July, I am the oldest person there.

Openly grimacing as if in pain, I float a question into the air 'That's a bit harsh isn't it?'

Jaz's face breaks into a massive grin. 'Don't worry mate. Ignore her – she's winding you up. You're looking pretty good. You're doing OK – for your age'.

Returning his grin, I move towards the bench. Without thinking, I scan the weights on the bar he has left for me. My assessment is I can begin with these and then build up over 4 sets. Leaning back flat on the bench, I flex my core and leg muscles to stabilise me and grasp the bar. My palms feel the coldness of the metal against the heat of my skin. The dimpled surface of the silver bar indents the pads of my fingers. I close my eyes, relax my grip slightly, let my arms hang and breathe gently.

The thumping beat of the music that pervades the gym recedes as I enter into stillness. An exhalation initiates the press. Through my palms the weight transfers down my triceps into my shoulders and chest as the muscles instantaneously start to stretch and hold. The bar descends touching my chest only to be propelled back upwards towards the sky. In this moment, my consciousness collapses into my pectoral muscles as they fire their straining message to my body that they are vibrant, alive and acting to order. Eleven more reps, they are flushed with blood, quivering to get the bar back into the rack. Linear time dissolves and becomes infused into my fibres. With each set, the weights get increased. The last press pushes me close to failure. On a shuddering, grunting completion there is no more power left. I am enveloped in the pleasure, the sensuality, of my burning pectorals. Lying on the bench, for a few seconds, I am fully present in my chest. I *am* my chest.

All too quickly, the rhythm, sounds and smells of the gym welcome me back. Standing I observe the happenings around me. All is recognisable and as it should be. Jaz is doing dips. If his triceps were to scream out for mercy from Lisa it would be no surprise. She is 'killing' him, and he pays for the pleasure of muscular development. There is ontological security in this mundaneness that comforts me. But then my mind flicks to what Jaz said: 'You're looking pretty good. You're doing OK – for your age'. I'm puzzled by what he meant. Looking pretty good to whom, compared to whom, using what criteria? Doing OK for what age? What are the markers of this age-related 'doing OK' in this setting? Is he judging me by how old I am or by how young I am not? In terms of the binary of youth and age that hierarchically arranges us in the gym, is my older body a disruption to the visual field of the dominant culture here tonight? Such questions intrigue me, but I understand they cannot be aired in the spaces of the gym tonight or any other night.

As part of my body maintenance routine and to alleviate the back pain that is my constant companion, my session concludes with some stretches in the matted area. The sensations and sensuality of elongating muscles and opening up joints is in direct contrast to that of pounding, compressing and contracting muscles. Lying on my back, I pull my knees to my chest and, holding them there with wrapped arms, begin to rock gently. The tension that inhabits the muscles of my lumbar spine resists me in an act of open defiance. Gradually, however, with the rhythmic rocking to-and-fro, they decide to join me in the motion and slowly let go of their tight hold. Their gentle release creates a warming glow deep in my lumbar region. This heat makes me acutely aware of a part of my body that too often, because it causes me pain, I try and force into submission via dissociation and objectification. Silently, I promise myself that, in the future, I will seek more of the pleasures of a stretching body.

Engrossed in my stretching, I did not notice the young woman join me on the mats. She is a regular trainer in the gym and works hard with the weights. The results are evident in the tight and toned body displayed in the close fitting attire she wears. We are on nodding terms, but I don't know her name or anything about her. Our only verbal communication is when I ask if she has finished with some equipment that I want to use. This is my level of knowledge about, and involvement with, almost all those who use this gym.

Glancing across at my companion of the mats, I recognise the slight grimace on her face as she manoeuvres her thighs up and down on the foam roller to massage the trigger points in her quadriceps to encourage the joys of myofascial release. From experience, I know this induces a radically different feeling to pumping weights and gentle stretching. As trigger points in the form of knotted muscles are compressed and released by limbs moving up and down the foam roller, an intense, electric burning sensation is momentarily induced followed by a wave of dispersing tension. The body part under focus is subjected to a sublime moment of pleasurable-pain and painful-pleasure that melt together as one.

I offer her an empathetic nod across the distance between us. She returns my communication in kind and, in so doing, acknowledges our unspoken understanding of quadriceps sensuality. Then a cold jab of shame, a sticky emotion, an intensely painful experience of the self by the self, freezes me in her momentary glance. In the rocking of my body my T-shirt has rolled up to expose a normally wrapped and hidden, rounded, soft belly. In its momentary brushing of my blushing skin the shame invites other emotions to attach itself to me in the form of humiliation, mortification and disgust. In that moment, I am fully present in my belly. I *am* my belly. Quickly, as these visceral emotions combine, the T-shirt is tucked back into my tracksuit bottoms. I vacate the matted area and head speedily to the changing rooms.

I can't remember when I first began to feel uncomfortable in the changing room of gyms or sports centres. As a young sportsman in school and then college my sinuous, athletic body was comfortable in the presence of other similarly muscled and finely tuned performance beings. Mine was the kind of body to have, the kind people wanted; my physical capital was high. Back then, I was not tyrannised by my reflections in the mirrors. Or was I? I can't be sure. Perhaps, this kind of tyranny can take many forms and my muscular frame served only to deflect attention away from a host of internal anxieties and contradictions I experienced. I do know that when my sports career was prematurely terminated by a back injury, I became less secure with my naked body in public spaces like the changing room. Over an 18-year period, after each of the three bouts of surgery on my lumbar spine, the doubts came seeping in about my capacity to maintain a disciplined and dominating body through various exercise regimes. These doubts and vulnerabilities clearly remain. They were confirmed in my deeply embodied reactions to that one glance a few minutes earlier from the young woman on the mat.

Right now, the small changing room that confines me is a space of abjection. I always arrive in my training gear. The locker is used only to secure my car keys and jacket. As I retrieve them, two young men in their mid-twenties stand talking as they dry themselves post-shower. Knowing the rules of visual engagement and the gaze in such places, I glance obliquely at their naked bodies. Their talk is of nutrition, the exercises they have just done and how aspects of their physique are responding to the regimes imposed on it. From my perspective, they are responding well. Their bodies are lean, cut and well proportioned. Both are tattooed, one more heavily than the other. The designs look good on their tight skin. As I slip on my jacket, one of them wraps a towel around his waist and steps towards the mirror over the washbasins. Without any sense of conceit he observes himself intently prior to pressing his palms together to flex his chest muscles.

'See, they're coming along', he says without diverting his gaze from the mirror.

This opinion is confirmed by his friend, who, staring directly at the contracted pectorals states, 'Yea, looking good'.

Both are comfortable in the changing room observing each other's body and making their aesthetic judgments on each. I seem invisible to them and quietly take my leave. Back home I shower in privacy. Drying myself in the bedroom I make the mistake of catching my reflection in the full length mirror. Jaz's words slip into my head: 'You're looking pretty good. You're doing OK – for your age'. The naked body that stares back at me does not believe a word of it and disdainfully removes itself from view to seek refuge in baggy clothing.

Reflections on the story

Reading the story above, I wonder what Jaz, Lisa and my brief companion on the mat, made of the fleeting moments we shared in that gym on that evening. I also wonder what you, the reader, make of the story from your own positioning. As Wellard (2014) points out, others occupying the same or similar places to the one I describe are likely to engage with, experience and understand themselves within it in very different ways depending on their age, gender, social class, sexual orientation, ethnicity/race, (dis)ability and religion. Therefore, the story I have constructed invites readings from a multiplicity of perspectives and would certainly benefit from a queer and crip reading.

I can also occupy the same place at other times and engage with, experience and understand myself within it in very different ways. For example, in contrast to the dominant feelings of shame and abjection I felt that night in the gym, on the following night, my sensory entanglements resulted in me experiencing the flow of intense and vibrant embodiment. For me, and many others, the gym can be heaven (liberating), it can be hell (repressive), or somewhere in between at any given moment (for example, see Sparkes, 2009, 2010, 2012). The gym as a territory may have fixed features (for example, where the squat racks are located), but the landscape within it is not fixed and stable. Rather, it is a fluid, dynamic place where multiple bodies come into being in various combinations. Deleuze and Guattari (1987) might describe it as an 'assemblage' that is composed of heterogeneous elements or objects that enter into relations with one another. These objects are not all of the same type. There are physical objects, happenings and events in the gym, but there are also regimes of signs, utterances and so on.

It is within the gym as a territory, a landscape and assemblage that my story unfolds. Here, I become situated and aware of myself as an aged and gendered being (amongst other things) as both a public body-object and a private subject-body in relation to others, like Jaz and Lisa, via the practices of *doing* my body while they simultaneously *do* theirs (Mol and Law, 2004). My experience of embodiment, therefore, is not a purely private affair, but is mediated by my continual interactions with other people and objects. As Blackman (2008: 105) might argue, our bodies in the gym that evening should not be conceived of as bounded and singular, but as open systems that 'connect to others, human and non-human, so that they are always unfinished and in a process of *becoming*'. She talks of multiplicity, movement, articulation, process and enactment for understanding the production of bodies across different sites, locations and practices. Blackman, along with others (for example, Laz, 2003), argues that all of us in the gym are individually and collectively, doing, enacting, accomplishing and performing our ages, masculinities and femininities in meaningful ways shaped by wider structural forces that permeate the air and our flesh.

Age, like gender, may not always be equally salient or meaningful in the same way in all situations. For example, all day before I visited the gym, my age was not foregrounded in my consciousness. Yet, clearly, it was an ever-present part of my landscape of self and my enactments as a university lecturer in an institutional setting where I interact daily with students several generations younger than me. The same might well be true for Lisa until the moment she looked around the gym and noticed, by drawing on culturally coded signs, categories of ageing and the feelings of inhabiting a particular body, that she was the 'second oldest' there. Her statement then draws my attention to my own ageing body as the 'oldest' in the gym. Age here is constituted in interaction and gains its meaning in the micro-dynamics of the event which, in turn, are shaped by the larger social forces that shape how we come to recognise and interpret the symbols, signs and feelings that take place in the gym. Gubrium and Holstein (2003), therefore, rightly criticise the commonly held perspective of ageing bodies as an omnipresent phenomenon when, in fact, in many everyday interactions it is sometimes 'invisible'. It is an object of experience whose visibility is determined by meaning-making action in specific contexts where the body is directly encountered in particular ways by self and others.

If the gym is taken as a place in which people *do* their age and gender (amongst other things) then questions can be raised about the resources that individuals draw on to accomplish these performances. A key resource I drew on in the gym that evening was my social and corporeal history of 59 years and its involvement with a range of body-reflexive practices that have been grounded in environments saturated by notions of hegemonic masculinity. Since my boyhood, these have quite literally shaped my body in terms of its muscular development, textures, sensualities, how I move in and use space and how I feel about inhabiting my body in relation to others that I interact with on a daily basis. For example, my immersion in contact sports as a 'star' player at secondary school and then college led to my 'habitus' (that is, a system of durable, transposable dispositions) to be developed within the confines of what Wellard (2009) calls 'expected and accepted sporting masculinity'. This is expressed and negotiated in the field of sport through bodily displays or performances involving aggression, competitiveness, power and assertiveness that have the effect of subordinating competing and alternative forms of masculinities as well as femininities.

This early involvement in sport as a domain of life was highly influential for me, along with many young men, in developing what Frank (2013) describes as an elective affinity for certain kinds of ideal body types (for example, disciplined and dominating) over others (for example, communicative). The disciplined body, according to Frank, defines itself primarily in actions of self-regimentation in the pursuit of control and predictability. The body in this process becomes an object, an 'it', to be worked on. The disciplined body is, therefore, dissociated from itself and is also monadic in it relations to other bodies.

Gyms, especially those that emphasise functional fitness and sport performance like the one I use, are places where predominantly young, disciplined (able)bodies are likely to flourish and feel at home. The process of ageing, however, as Twigg (2004) reminds us, forces an engagement with physiology in ways that are likely to prove problematic in relation to this type of body given that athletic performance, in 'absolute' terms, is likely to decrease over time. In this regard, Eman (2012) speaks of 'capability-age'. This involves a reading of age through physical capabilities, which is largely enabled through practicing sports and physical activities that make bodily experiences more accessible. Capability-age is assessed mainly though comparisons of current physical experiences with previous abilities and with the abilities of others. In her study of the role of sports in making sense of the process of growing old, Eman found that these comparisons differed by gender, with men focusing primarily on their athletic results (for example, kilograms bench pressed in the gym) and women on their performance. For men, if their measured results deteriorated, this was perceived as a sign of oldness. Eman notes that physical control and competence functions as physical capital for athletically active older men, both in a gendered and ageing context. She also points out that athletic men rely on their appearance to maintain their more youthful self-images in the process of ageing.

Given the characteristics of the disciplined body described earlier, it is likely that this body type will be both attracted and threatened by the enactment of capability-ageing. The attraction comes with what Eman (2012) calls the semblance of objectivity in evaluating themselves and others because it is visible and quantifiable which lends itself to schedules and regimes of training, and in the gym by the reflection of the owner's body in the mirror. The threat is that, by definition, physical performance levels as indicated by these objective measurements are likely to decrease as one ages, as is one's body shape and texture. These decreases are likely to be interpreted by the disciplined, ageing male body in the gym in relation to the narrative habitus of the individual involved.

For Frank (2010: 52–53) the narrative habitus involves the embedding of stories in bodies so that some stories are heard, immediately and intuitively, as belonging to a certain body and self. For Frank, this kind of habitus is a 'disposition to hear some stories as those one ought to listen to, ought to repeat on appropriate occasions, and ought to be guided by'. It describes the embodied sense of attraction, indifference or repulsion that people feel in response to stories, which leads them to define some as *for us* or not for us. Narrative habitus, therefore, 'is the unchosen force in any choice to be interpellated by a story, and the complementary rejection of the interpellation that other stories would effect if a person were caught up in them'. Such choices take place within specific cultures and subcultures that provide people with a menu, or repertoire, of narrative forms and contents from which they selectively draw in an effort to line up their lived experience with the kinds of stories available to organise and express it to their self and others. Significantly, the dominant narrative in Western cultures associated with ageing, which becomes intensified in sporting subcultures, remains that of 'decline' (Phoenix and Sparkes, 2007, 2008, 2009).

The notion of decline signals a reduction in control over one's corporeality both in terms of the public body-object and the private subject-body. Significantly, as Frank (2013) notes, the disciplined body experiences its greatest crisis in loss of control. When faced with this crisis, it seeks to reassert predictability through therapeutic regimes, such as training with weights. Against this backdrop, my story from the gym illustrates the vulnerability of the disciplined body as it ages, the impact this can have on such bodies to perform specific forms of masculinity in public places, and both the affect and effect this can have on the person in the process.

My story also raises questions about narrative imaginings. We could ask how might a different kind of ideal body type, drawing on different narrative resources, have made sense of events in the gym that evening? What if the body I inhabited then had been more of the communicative type described by Frank (2013)? This kind of body, (a) accepts its contingency as normative and as part of the fundamental contingency of life, (b) understands that for all its resilience, it is fragile with breakdown built into it and (c) recognises that the bodily predictability, so desired and required of the disciplined body, if not the exception, should be regarded as exceptional. Accordingly, the communicative body is fully associated with itself and is dyadic in its relationship with others.

As an ageing man, I am left pondering the possibilities and potentials of myself and others like me, of inhabiting a more communicative body in the gym. What might this mean for how I perform and interpret the masculinities that I embody in this and other places? Such a body, that does not fear contingency but embraces it, would seem more attuned and aligned with the multiplicity, movement and articulations that Blackman (2008) spoke of in the unfinished process of becoming in places as assemblages and shifting landscapes. As part of this unfinished process of becoming, shifts in the narrative habitus become possible so that stories about ageing that have previously been left to float by in the river-of-not-for me (Frank, 2010) can now be seriously considered and gradually embedded in the flesh. This embedding of different stories, acting as counter-narratives, can alter the experiential dynamics of ageing and offer a corporeal resource for challenging the tyranny of the decline narrative.

Expanding or shifting one's narrative habitus is, however, as Frank (2010) acknowledges, no easy task. Part of the problem lies in finding suitable counter-narratives. One might suspect that a suitable candidate here would be the 'successful ageing' narrative as described by Lamb (2014: 45). This narrative has the following characteristics: an emphasis on agency and control, the individual self/body as a project to be worked on, the maintenance of independence, the maintenance of productive activity (physical, cognitive and social) and finally, the notion of 'permanent personhood'. These characteristics, both individually and collectively, have strong resonances with the disciplined body and its desire for predictability and control via self-regimentation, and the gym would be an ideal place for this disciplined, successfully ageing body to be performed on a regular basis. This is particularly so in relation to the notion of 'permanent personhood' that contains a vision of the *ideal* person as an *ageless* self who does not really age at all in late life, but rather maintains the self of one's earlier years, 'while avoiding or denying processes of decline, mortality and human transience'.

As Lamb (2014) points out, however, while the successful ageing narrative may contain inspirational elements, in some ways it is actually counterproductive. This is because, as she vividly illustrates, this narrative in Western cultures over-emphasises independence, prolonging life and 'declining to decline', at the expense of coming to meaningful terms with age-related changes, situations of (inter)dependence, possibilities of frailty and the condition of human transience. In the face of inevitable bodily or cognitive impairments, this sets up a situation of inbuilt 'failure', embarrassment or loss of social personhood for those involved. Against this, Lamb argues that the successful ageing narrative needs to change by recognising and incorporating the notion of meaningful decline as a valid dimension of ageing and personhood. Such a change would connect well to the characteristics of the communicative body described by Frank (2013) and open up productive possibilities for the ageing body in the gym and other physical activity settings. This said, as I hope the story offered in this chapter illustrates, there is much to be done to transform these possibilities into realities by changing the narrative habitus and generating different narrative imaginings of how ageing, masculine bodies are performed and experienced in physical activity settings.

References

Blackman L (2008) *The Body*. Oxford: Berg.
Deleuze G and Guattari, F (1987) *A Thousand Plateaus: Capitalism and Schizophrenia*. New York: Continuum.
Eman J (2012) The role of sport in making sense of growing old. *Journal of Aging Studies* 26: 467–475.
Frank A (2010). *Letting Stories Breathe: A Socio-Narratology*. Chicago: University of Chicago Press.
Frank A (2013) *The Wounded Storyteller* (2nd edition). Chicago: University of Chicago Press.
Gubrium J and Holstein J (2003) The everyday visibility of the ageing body. In: C Faircloth (ed) *Ageing Bodies*. New York: Altamira Press, pp. 205–227.
Gullette M (2003) From life storytelling to age autobiography. *Journal of Aging Studies* 17: 101–111.
Lamb S (2014) Permanent personhood and meaningful decline? toward a critical anthropology of successful aging. *Journal of Aging Studies* 29: 41–52.
Laz C (2003) Age embodied. *Journal of Aging Studies* 17: 503–519.
Mol A and Law J (2004) Embodied action, enacted bodies: the example of hypoglycaemia. *Body and Society* 10: 43–62.
Phoenix C and Sparkes A (2007) Sporting bodies, ageing, narrative mapping and young team athletes: an analysis of possible selves. *Sport, Education and Society* 12: 1–17.

Phoenix C and Sparkes A (2008) Athletic bodies and aging in context: the narrative construction of experienced and anticipated selves in time. *Journal of Aging Studies* 22: 211–221.

Phoenix C and Sparkes A (2009) Being Fred: big stories, small stories and the accomplishment of a positive ageing identity. *Qualitative Research* 9: 219–236.

Shirani F (2013) The spectre of the wheezy Dad: masculinity, fatherhood and ageing. *Sociology* 47, 1104–1119.

Sparkes A (2009) Ethnography and the senses: challenges and possibilities. *Qualitative Research in Sport, Exercise and Health* 1: 21–35.

Sparkes A (2010) Performing the ageing body and the importance of place: some brief autoethnographic moments. In: B Humberstone (ed) *'When I am old...' Third Age and Leisure Research: Principles and Practice*. Eastbourne, UK: Leisure Studies Association, pp. 21–32.

Sparkes A (2012) Fathers and sons: in bits and pieces. *Qualitative Inquiry* 18: 167–178.

Twigg J (2004) The body, gender, and age: feminist insights in social gerontology. *Journal of Aging Studies* 18: 59–73.

Wellard I (2009) *Sport, Masculinities and the Body*. London: Routledge.

Wellard I (2014) *Sport, Fun and Enjoyment*. London: Routledge.

14
Ageing Women Still Play Games: (Auto)ethnographic Research in a Fitness Intervention

Gertrud Pfister and Verena Lenneis

Introduction

Fitness and youth may have been assets in all cultures and societies. However, with the great advances in medicine and the proliferation of human improvement technologies, a youthful appearance and a healthy body seem to be the obligation of dutiful citizens. With the help of numerous means of enhancement ranging from diet to surgery the dream of eternal youth and perfect health seems to be within reach. Among the multitude of health-related 'best practices' physical activities and sport have a special significance. They have been recognised as a powerful 'anti-ageing medicine' and are highly recommended as a remedy for numerous problems and afflictions, among them diabetes and obesity, as well as menopausal symptoms and health problems connected with ageing.

Currently numerous scholars are exploring the impact of physical activities and sports on various ageing processes: among them the scientists working at the Centre for Team Sport and Health at the University of Copenhagen. They are investigating the effects of ball games, in particular of football and floorball, on certain health parameters of the participants. Among their 'guinea pigs' are old men as well as groups of ageing women, even though team sports are considered activities for young people, more exactly young men. Among the 6,040 members of the Danish Floorball Federation, 81% are boys and men, and 41% are less than 18 years of age.[1]

This chapter focuses on my (GP) and other women's experiences with playing floorball in a fitness intervention, as well as on the opportunities and challenges they encountered during their participation in activities which did not 'fit' their age or their gender. How did they cope with playing a game which they had never tried before; how did they handle being part of a team and how did they fare in a group of women whom they had met for the first time at the start of the project? These questions have been raised in a research project evaluating an intervention in which 23 ageing women (including myself) played floorball twice a week.

Preliminary thoughts on sport, sports sciences and ageing

First encounters with the floorball project

I work at the Institute of Nutrition, Exercise and Sports, and I am used to seeing young and fit sports students running, throwing the javelin or playing football out of my window. It is a pleasure to watch these young men and women competing in mixed teams; they are motivated, highly skilled and so eager to score a goal. When I was a sports student many years ago, women did not learn to play football, and now I am too old to begin with a team sport – at least, this was what I thought when I observed these young people.

Being surrounded by all these athletic students, I was a bit surprised when I saw older women with sports bags entering our gym hall. One hour later they came out again, chattering, laughing, sweating and looking rather tired. I wondered in which programme they were participating, what kind of exercises they were doing and why they were looking so drained and dishevelled. Some days later I followed them into the hall and saw them playing floorball, a 'fast-paced, exciting, safe and low-cost type of indoor hockey'[2] which is very popular in Denmark. The women played on a small field surrounded by low banks which let the ball bounce back. The hockey sticks are made of plastic and the goal is hip high. Obviously the players were having a lot of fun; they laughed, shouted and clapped each other on the shoulder when one of them scored a goal.

The women were middle-aged; later I learned that they were between 45 to 55 years of age, that is, much younger than me. They were of all shapes and sizes, and some carried quite a lot of weight around with them. A small blond player looked quite diminutive beside a tall woman with a dark ponytail towering over her, but despite the advantage of being tall, she did not manage to get the puck when the small Dane darted off. The women all wore heart rate monitors, which indicated that they were participating in one of the numerous experiments carried out by my colleagues working in the area of sports physiology. What were they researching this time? Why did they let women of this age play a game?

An instructor cheered them on, shouted advice and finally whistled to signal a break. The players sat down; some even sprawled on the floor, and some got their water bottles to have a drink or fetched their towels to dry their sweating faces. This provided the opportunity to talk to the instructor, a student whom I knew from one of my courses – and he explained that this was a project of the Centre for Team Sport and Health.

The Centre for Team Sport and Health and the floorball intervention

The Centre for Team Sport and Health is a research institute at the University of Copenhagen with the 'mission to create a significant difference in the health of the Danish population'.[3] The physiologists who were conducting this study considered ageing as a 'problem' because of the hormonal changes and their effects on several physiological processes.

They wanted to explore the specific effects of exercises on physiological parameters of women before and after the menopause (see Nyberg et al., 2014). Their first results made headlines: 'Floorball compensates for the loss of oestrogen'.[4]

Why floorball? Although the effect of physical activities does not depend on the type of the activity, many fitness programmes have proved to be useless because the participants, jogging on a running belt or pedalling on an indoor cycle, get bored after a while and give up. Letting the people play games seemed to be an alternative to traditional health-sport activities. Inspired by this insight, some colleagues experimented with 'football fitness', that is, football with simple rules played on a small field. The success of this new form of playing encouraged them to found a Centre for Team Sport and Health. The 'floorball women' participated in one of the Centre's favourite projects, not least because they were a new target group and because other colleagues doubted whether women of this age could engage in a ball game.

Ageing as a woman who loves sport

Working at a sports institute as an older woman has both positive and negative sides. I love sport, and I like to be able to train at my working place and to be able to do research about a large variety of sport-related topics. However, from the perspective of sports scientists, ageing causes problems, as mentioned above. In particular physiologists have a 'deficit' perspective when they talk and deal with older people, and in this regard older women (not least because of decreased oestrogen levels and the loss of their 'reproductive functions') are evaluated even worse than older men, and it is no fun for an ageing woman like myself to be confronted with lectures and discussions about the decaying bodies of older women.

The medical view of ageing women complies with and contributes to 'youthism' in modern societies, that is, the glorification of youth and the pursuit of a young(-looking), slim and trimmed body (for example, Clarke and Griffin, 2008). Both the idealisation of youth on the one hand and the stereotypes about ageing on the other are gendered: women seemingly lose an important asset, that is, a youthful appearance, whereas men may still be considered attractive because competence and power are important features of their image. However, with the help of current enhancement technologies, eternal youth – at least with regard to appearance – seems possible. There are also various means, from medication to cosmetic surgery, of counteracting some of the changes during the climacteric. The rise of anti-ageing industries is a consequence of the pathologisation of the menopause and of ageing. However, ageing also has positive consequences, for example, the cessation of menstruation. Representative studies in many countries have shown that happiness is positively linked with ageing with a peak of happiness at 69 (Gregoire, 2014). But the positive sides of ageing seldom make the headlines and do not change ageism.

I often experience the 'deficit gaze' directed at older women, and I am confronted with youthism when I see advertisements for beauty products or when I read about the costs of healthcare caused by an ageing population. However, getting older has not changed my self-image – at least as long as I do not look in the mirror or feel the gaze of others. What do they see? Do they still perceive me as competent and strong, able to play games? Or do they see the 'mask of ageing' contributing to the invisibility of me as an ageing woman? The promises and threats of the enhancement society, that is, the possibility of beautification and the threat of stigmatisation, may trigger different reactions: attempts to be 'forever young' or to resist the 'youth codes' and attempt to fight ageism instead of ageing.

Theoretical considerations and methods

The interest in ageing, our questions, our 'gaze' and our interpretations are guided not only by everyday experiences, but also by theoretical assumptions. Youthism and healthism (Crawford, 1980, 2006) as dominant ideologies in modern societies and gender as a social arrangement as well as a self-presentation in interactions embedded in subjectivities (Connell, 2002; Lorber, 1994) have already been addressed in the preceding paragraphs.

The context of our research, the bio-medical paradigms of the project and in general the 'strength of biomedicine in the current discursive space within the field of ageing' (Dumas and Turner, 2013: 68) drew our attention to the deficit perspective, which were central themes in the physiologists' discussions about the intervention and its participants. Menopause and ageing were considered as problems. Drawing on Foucault, Katz (1996) uses the concept of problematisation to emphasise the contradictory discourses and reactions to the 'problem' of ageing in Western cultures. According to this approach, anti-ageing strategies such as fitness interventions seem to generate 'contempt towards ageing bodies' and suggest at the same time that ageing is avoidable (Dumas and Turner, 2013: 68).

From a Bourdieusian perspective (Bourdieu, 1984), the intervention can be understood as a body-maintenance technique which provides or enhances 'physical capital' in a period of time when the value of this capital is expected to decrease.

Using autoethnography, we chose a form and method of research and writing that aimed to describe and analyse personal experience in order to understand discourses and practices embedded in the specific context, in this case the context of the intervention (for a similar approach see, for example, Griffin, 2012). Autoethnographic studies give voices to the research participants and allow and even require subjective perspectives and judgements of the researchers in order to uncover and understand the 'situated knowledge' and the experiences of the participants. In addition, the second author conducted in-depth individual interviews with 17 women, which contained extensive narrative parts. The accounts given in the interviews complemented the insights gained during the fieldwork and helped to uncover the aims, experiences and evaluations of the women. The combination of these methods allowed a triangulation, that is, the validation of interpretations by cross-checking the information.

Experiences and interpretations – fieldwork

The first field notes

Thursday, 28 March 2013: participant observation during the floorball intervention with 'pre- and post-menopausal women'. Place: sports hall, Nørre Allé, 16.00 to 17.15.

Already in my training outfit, I walk over to the sports hall. The instructor arrives together with me. A tall and athletic young PhD student, he brings the sticks and the balls, as well as other equipment. We talk briefly about his project, and I find out that the participants are 45 to 55 years old, half of them 'post-menopausal' and the other half in the control group. Can I really play with these 'young' women?

One after the other, the participants arrive. They change into their sports outfits, register and get a heart rate monitor, which they fix on their bodies. I observe them secretly; they look fit and do not seem to be ageing at all. Again I feel a bit insecure; I do not want to make a fool of myself. In addition, I am worried about floorball, a sport which I have never played. Will I be able to strike the ball? Or will I miss it all the time and become a laughing stock? And the others – would they swing their sticks clumsily and perhaps even hit me with them? Why do we not wear helmets?

One woman begins to put the barriers in place along both sides of the 'floorball field'. These knee-high white plastic barriers make the ball bounce back and prevent it from 'escaping' – which makes the game fast; there's no waiting until the ball is brought back from the other side of the hall. I help the woman and ask her name. Now I know at least one of the group. The instructor briefly introduces me as a sociologist, but the women are not curious and those who arrive later are not informed about my role at all. This is just great – I want to be treated like everybody else.

During the warming-up and in the breaks I look at the different women and wonder which of them belong to the 'pre-menopausal' group. They do not look very different, and I wonder how old they think I am. I am sure that I am much older than they are, but I hope that they do not notice or at any rate do not care. But they do not seem to be interested in me or my reasons for being here. But I am curious: why are they taking part in this programme and why did they choose the floorball intervention? Because they know this sport or because it is more fun than fitness exercises? Do they play other sports? Some of them may want to get rid of a few kilos, but overweight women are only a small minority here. Do they want to get or keep fit? Why? No doubt some want to do something for their health. Given the ubiquitous health discourses in the country, they must have heard about the health benefits of physical activities. Do they have medical problems and issues, perhaps as a consequence of the menopause, and do they hope to overcome these problems by exercising? In spite of these reflections, I function like all the others: we run, hit or miss the ball and sweat profusely.

After half an hour we are ready for the 'real thing'. The instructor gives us vests of different colours and forms three teams. Two play while one has a break. The game begins.

This was the first time that I had played floorball, so I did not handle the ball very well, but I tried hard and ran after all balls, which made me quite successful – some women even asked me if I had played before. I was very proud and had suddenly forgotten about my age.

During the break I have time to observe. The women are very different: tall and thin, tall and heavy; most are 'normal' as regards size and weight; a few are small or tiny. They have long hair in pony tails; middle-long hair held back with a hair band; another one has short and curly hair. Colours vary a lot: grey, blond, black, reddish or brown mixed with grey. Most of them are wearing black long trousers and tops of different colours – no fancy outfits, just functional clothes. They play with enthusiasm; sometimes they even perform body checks – mostly unintentionally. The two tall and heavy women are the goal keepers, and it is difficult to score as there is not a lot of space for the ball to slip past them. The others run a lot, trying to stick to an opponent and prevent her from getting the ball or trying to get rid of a 'shadow' in order to get a free shot.

There are cries of joy or anger when the ball is in the goal; sometimes the scorer gets a high five but nobody counts the goals. In a break we discuss which team is winning. We cannot agree upon the score, but it does not matter. This lack of concern about the outcome of the game, though, does not prevent us from trying hard and giving our best (which in my case is mostly running and snatching the ball from opponents who do not expect my coming from the other side of the field).

After the six minutes I am covered in sweat and so are the others. We are happy to have a 'time out', and another team takes our place on the field. Some players just lie down gasping for air while others sit on their towels. Everybody drinks water. When we have – more or less – recovered, we have to enter the field again.

Soon, too soon, the game is over. I am not aware that we have played for more than half an hour but I realise, when the final whistle blows, that I am utterly exhausted.

During the stretching there is a lot of joking – some of it about men. They discuss, for example, what kind of men women need and agree that every woman needs three men: one for sex, one to earn money and one as a companion for cultural events. There is consensus that one man cannot fulfil all three requirements.

Others add witty comments, and we all laugh a lot. Only the instructor is silent. Then everybody is in a hurry: home, family and dinner are waiting, and some have a rendezvous at a restaurant. They go into the shower rooms; I walk to my office, where I had left my street clothes. I feel many muscles that I did not even know existed. I am proud that I was able to keep up with the other women. Cycling home, I decide to continue with the training programme on Saturday.

PS: Already half an hour later I have terribly aching muscles, and I feel my old age!!!

Reflections and questions

The observations, the informal talks and also the reflections about my own experiences raised the following interconnected questions: Why did the women take part in the floorball training programme? What prevented most of them from dropping out (which occurs frequently in such projects)? What did they consider to be the benefits of participating? Was keeping fit and young one of their motives?

The field notes of the following training sessions provide some answers. They contain not only my experiences with the game (I improved my play), but also the encounters with the other women: the stories about their jobs and their families, the exchange of recipes and information about good restaurants in the locker room, the laughing and chatting under the shower, the joy when their team played well, complaints about aching muscles or the celebration of a goal with high fives. Many women loved the physicality of the game and the excitement of scoring and winning. During the game we acted as young women, but afterwards we felt our age. Most of us had small problems – bruises, a hurting hip or an aching muscle – but we joked about them.

An important topic in the locker room was the physiological tests, for example the pain of muscle biopsies as well as the results. The women were very interested in their data and also in physiological changes as a result of the intervention. Their remarks about the tests and their outcomes revealed not only a certain degree of medical knowledge, but also their concern about their health, their fear of getting/looking old and their willingness to comply with healthism. A few women also hoped to lose weight.

The field notes also indicate that the women enjoyed very much being a member of this group and playing in a team, as well as the fact that playing triggered a flow element and that mastering the game conveyed pride and increased self-esteem. The relatively wide age differences did not play a role: as the oldest participant by far, I felt accepted and forgot about my age. There was a certain 'social order' in the group, with some women having more influence than others, and there was even an 'official' spokeswoman. However, there were no outsiders – which for me was also a reason for coming to the training sessions. These questions were also raised in the interviews and answered in a reflected and in-depth way.

Interviews

Semi-structured interviews with guidelines took up the issues presented above and provided information about the motives and experiences of the floorball players.

The interviews showed that the participants were well informed about the health benefits of physical activities, in particular for older women. Some hoped to alleviate menopausal symptoms by participating in the floorball project. All of them had, at least to some degree, internalised the prevailing health discourses in Danish society, which emphasise the individual's responsibility to adopt a healthy life-style (see, for example, Scocozza, 2009; Vallgårda, 2009). Although most of them had participated in sports in various phases of their lives (though none of them had tried to play floorball before), they had adopted a sedentary life-style and were glad about the project and having the opportunity to be physically active (and comply with the official health recommendations. They also told us that they were in a phase of life in which people had to cope with illness and diseases and also had to reflect on ways of preventing disease. The fact that there was a coach and a team waiting for them provided the necessary incentive, or even obligation, to take part regularly.

In addition, the 'community of players' had a strong appeal for the participants. They appreciated the fact that all participants were women of a similar age, that none of them had any previous experience of playing floorball and that there were no large age differences in the group. They were all ageing, and the floorball training programme offered them a 'safe' space where they could compete amongst equally skilled players and did not have to worry about not being able to keep up with the others.

For many women the 'flow element' of playing was the most important incentive to come to the training sessions. Interviewees described this feeling as follows: 'I think it [the training] is both exciting and exhausting. At the same time it's also fun. ... It's a lot of fun. It's like you're a child again and playing. You forget your age', or, 'I've had several moments where I felt like I was 100% present on the playing field. You know, such a moment where you think, damn it, how great this is'. Another woman described playing as a form of 'meditation': 'You forget about everything and clear your head. ... So it's really a great feeling to play team sports'.

Although the players trained hard, the training was not experienced as work but as fun: 'I've never experienced this before – where I was drenched in sweat and totally out of breath, but so engaged that I don't notice at all how tired I am'. Two other women added: 'You are exhausted afterwards and sometimes I guess that you push yourself too hard, but you don't really realise it until afterwards. While I am playing, I don't feel that it's exercise'. The benefits of playing a game are highlighted by an interviewee who compared floorball training with training in a fitness centre: 'When you play floorball, you don't really notice that time passes. You are doing something, which is fun. Hard, but also fun. Going to the fitness centre is of course also hard, but it's not fun for sure'.

Pride, self-image and fitness

In part because the women had not had any recent encounters with sports and also did not have any great sports-related skills, playing floorball provided immediate success experiences, even for unskilled participants: 'I have never tried to do team sports before. Never! I don't come from a family where people have done sports. I've never experienced a situation where it wasn't myself I had to focus on. Now I don't have to focus on myself, but on the game, the ball and the others'.

In addition, the participants felt not only an improvement in their playing skills, but also a considerable increase in their fitness. When the intervention ended, many women decided to continue to play, and they still do so today, changing their role from research objects to subjects who in some ways connect their desire for health with their desire for fun.

Conclusion

Observations and interviews provided excellent insights into the backgrounds, motives and experiences of ageing women who participated in a physiological intervention and discovered that they were able to participate in ball games. Influenced by the health discourses in Danish society, they expected training to be hard work and found out that it could also be fun. The flow element of playing, the good relations among the participants and the obligation to come to the training sessions because the instructor and the other women were waiting contributed to the success of this project. From the perspective of the physiologists, success meant that they were able to conduct their tests before and after the project. But from the perspective of the participants, success meant that they experienced themselves as capable, responsible and pro-active individuals and that they were able to continue to play because they loved the game.

I have learned – and I think the other women too – that age is relative, depending on the situation, and that mastering a task and having fun with others does not depend on age.

However, it must also be taken into consideration that, according to a socio-demographic analysis, the participants in this study had a relatively high socio-economic status and a close network of social support. Whether, or to what extent, these results can be repeated in projects with other groups is therefore an open question. We must also bear in mind that ethnographic fieldwork and interviews only allow concrete insight into the actions and the interrelations of a specific group in a specific situation. However, the results provide knowledge that may put forward hypotheses and be used as a point of departure for further studies.

I have to confess that I did not continue to play floorball, firstly because of overlapping schedules. But then I had lost contact with the women, and in addition I was afraid that they had become too good for me to be able to play with them any longer.

Acknowledgements

The study was supported by Nordea-fonden, Denmark.

Notes

1. http://www.floorball.dk/Nyheder/Nyheder/2012/3/Medlemsindberetning%20 2011.aspx
2. http://www.floorballpro.com/shop/pages.php?pageid=17
3. See the information on the website http://www.holdspil.ku.dk/english/
4. Holdspil kompenserer for tab af østrogen [Team sports compensates for the loss of estrogen] (21 February 2014). Retrieved from http://nyheder.ku.dk/alle_nyheder/2014/02/holdspil-kompenserer-for-tab-af-oestrogen/

References

Bourdieu P (1984) *Distinction: A Social Critique of the Judgement of Taste*. Cambridge, MA: Harvard University Press.
Clarke LH and Griffin M (2008) Visible and invisible ageing: beauty work as a response to ageism. *Ageing and Society* 28(5): 653–674.
Connell RW (2002) *Gender*. Cambridge: Polity.
Crawford R (1980) Healthism and the medicalization of everyday life. *International Journal of Health Services* 10: 365–388.

Crawford R (2006) Health as a meaningful social practice. *Health* 10: 401–420.
Dumas A and Turner BS (2013) Statecraft and soulcraft: Foucault on prolonging life. In: WC Cockerham (ed) *Medical Sociology on the Move: New Directions in Theory*. Dordrecht, The Netherlands: Springer, pp. 61–81.
Gregoire C (2014) Here's scientific proof that life gets better as you get older. *The Huffington Post*. Available at: http://www.huffingtonpost.com/2014/04/10/scientific-proof-that-the_n_5110179.html (accessed October 2014).
Griffin MB (2012) *Health Consciousness, Running and Female Bodies: An Ethnographic Study of 'Active Ageing'*. Unpublished Thesis (Ph.D.). Exeter, UK: University of Exeter.
Katz S (1996) *Disciplining Old Age: The Formation of Gerontological Knowledge*. Charlottesville, VA: University Press of Virginia.
Lorber J (1994) *Paradoxes of Gender*. New Haven, CT: Yale University Press.
Nyberg MP, Seidelin K, Anderson TR, Overby NN, Hellsten Y and Bangsbo J (2014) Biomarkers of vascular function in premeanopausal and recent post-menopausal women of similar age. *American Journal of Physiology* 306(7): R510–R517.
Scocozza L (2009) Folkesundhed eller moralsk oprustning? [Public health or moral rearmament?] In: S Glasdam and I Axelsen (eds) *Folkesundhed: i et Kritisk Perspektiv*. Copenhagen: Nyt Nordisk Forlag, pp. 54–66.
Vallgårda S (2009) Sundhedspolitik i de skandinaviske lande [Health policy in the Scandinavian countries]. In: S Glasdam and I Axelsen (eds). *Folkesundhed: i et Kritisk Perspektiv*. Copenhagen: Nyt Nordisk Forlag, pp. 166–187.

15
Physical Activity among Older Adults with Visual Impairment: Considerations for Ageing Well with Sight Loss

Meridith Griffin

Introduction

Almost 2 million people in the UK are living with sight loss that has a significant impact on their daily lives, and every day approximately 100 more people begin to lose their sight (Fight for Sight, 2013). This phenomenon is increasingly linked to age, with 1 in 9 people aged 60+ in the UK currently living with sight loss. Research shows that visually impaired older adults, in general, have poorer general health than the sighted population (Jones et al., 2009). Visual impairment is also a significant risk factor for additional medical conditions as a result of activity limitations and participation restrictions (Crews and Campbell, 2001).

Whilst not a panacea or a simplistic anti-ageing strategy (see Tulle, 2008), being physically active can help improve health and prevent secondary medical conditions. For example, physically active older adults have lower risk of disease including dementia and have higher levels of physical and cognitive function, psychological well-being and independence than inactive older adults (Department of Health (DoH), 2013). Despite such benefits, very few older adults – and even fewer older adults with a disability of any kind – meet the minimum amounts of activity recommended for health (30 minutes of at least moderate physical activity on five or more days per week) (Craig et al., 2008; DoH, 2013; Department for Work and Pensions (DWP), 2013; Sport England, 2011, 2013).

This chapter summarises the findings of a collaborative qualitative research project that aimed to increase the knowledge of physical activity among older people with acquired sight loss later in life by (a) exploring their individual experiences of physical activity and (b) identifying ways in which participation in physical activity can be facilitated and/ or prevented. Insights from this work go some way toward providing an evidence base with examples of good and poor practice, which can be used to inform policy and programming regarding the promotion of physical activity among older people with sight loss. Moreover, the research points to several areas for future research that have the potential to develop knowledge with regards to improving commercial enterprise and service delivery in this area.

Context and conceptual background

Both social gerontology and disability studies tend to overlook the experience of ageing with disabilities (Kennedy and Minkler, 1998; Priestley and Rabiee, 2002). That said, in the gerontological literature there are an abundance of studies on impairment in late life. These tend to take a functionalist perspective that views impairment as a result of an age-based process of decline, rather than exploring disability as an *intersecting* location of experience (Raymond et al., 2014; Townsend, 2007). Disability studies also tend to overlook the process of ageing. Although strong in a critique of ableism and access, disability studies stress the commonality of oppression for people with impairments, thereby obscuring how disabling societies differentially affect individuals throughout their life course (Priestley, 2003). Disability studies have also been criticised for being largely disembodied (Freund, 2001; Hughes and Paterson, 1997; Paterson and Hughes, 1999).

Depending on the specific condition, age-related sight loss can be gradual, with deterioration occurring over time, or very sudden. In addition, the level or degree of sight loss can be complete or partial, affecting either visual acuity or visual field. These variations make for very different lived experiences – but regardless, the shift in sensory capacity represents a disruption to the embodied ageing process. It necessitates adaptation to activities of daily living as well as supplemental activities including leisure and recreation. Physical activity is often placed in this category, requiring the older adult with acquired sight loss to adapt pre-existing activities (if applicable) or learn new activities should they desire to do so. This involves navigating a new embodied experience, something made possible with structural and emotional support and guidance from significant others, rehabilitation officers, and blind or partially sighted peers. Availability of these and other resources is not equally distributed, nor does each older adult cope with their sight loss in the same way.

Taking the perspective then that visual impairment is both social and embodied, research in this area must extend its focus beyond a structural or social model approach that attends to the socio-structural barriers that serve to exclude and restrict people with impairments. This is warranted because the psycho-emotional dimensions of disabled people's lives are deliberately not attended to within the social model (Goodley, 2011; Smith and Sparkes, 2012; Thomas, 2007). As such, we are left with an inadequate understanding of the lived experience of older adults with sight loss and the complex ways in which they may be restricted from engaging in physical activity. In light of this inadequate understanding of disability, and recent criticisms of the social model (see Goodley, 2011), one possible way forward is to consider the social relational model of disability as described by Thomas (2007).

The social relational model describes disability as 'a form of social oppression involving the social imposition of restrictions of activity on people with impairments and the socially engendered undermining of their psycho-emotional well-being' (Thomas, 2007: 73). Conceptualised this way, this model uniquely extends the social model by proposing that it is not just the physical environment that restricts people's physical activity (that is, structural disablism). The social relational model also deliberately proposes that restrictions of activity arise when a person's psycho-emotional wellbeing is damaged. One way this damage can occur, and thus activities restricted, is through interactions with other people.

Recent publications indicate that ageing has emerged as a new focus within disability studies (Jeppsson Grassman and Witaker, 2013). Given that the 'greying' of the population will result in a greater number of older people with disabilities (and visual impairment specifically), there is a need to link social gerontology and disability studies – and to focus therein on the embodied, lived experience of older adults with sight loss in order to best understand the complexity with which they experience the world in general, and physical activity in particular. Certainly, meaningful changes to activity levels and subsequent health and wellbeing cannot be made until the lived experience of older adults with sight loss is better understood.

Methods and methodology

After gaining university ethical approval for the study, participants were recruited using a purposive sampling strategy that was informed by maximum variation sampling in order to capture a diverse range of views (Sparkes and Smith, 2014). The inclusion criteria were (a) adults with acquired sight loss (that is, non-congenital) and (b) aged 60+. Participants were recruited from 3 different geographical areas in England (the South West, the Midlands and London) and from a range of settings via local sight loss organisations and advertisements in talking newspapers. Upon expressing interest in the research, prospective participants were asked to fill out a biographical questionnaire (with assistance if required) wherein they confirmed their age and self-identified their current type and level of vision loss. Categories for these self-reports of visual impairment were drawn from the English Longitudinal Study of Ageing regarding visual impairment (ELSA, 2013). Recruitment of each participant group continued until data saturation was achieved and there were no more emergent patterns in the data (Green and Thorogood, 2009). The result was a recruited sample of 48 visually impaired people comprising of 24 males and 24 females who (via self-report) identified a variety of activity levels – from being inactive to highly active.

Participants took part in semi-structured interviews in a location of their choosing – primarily this was in their own homes and occasionally in a local coffee shop or quiet meeting place. Interviews were digitally recorded, and all data were subsequently transcribed verbatim. Data were analysed using an inductive thematic analysis involving the systematic organisation, description and interpretation of the key patterns (themes) within the data set (Braun and Clark, 2006).

Findings

From the thematic analysis, 2 broad themes were identified: (1) Health characteristics and (2) Accessibility and opportunity. Within each theme there are several contributing sub-themes, describing both barriers and facilitators to participation in physical activity among older adults with sight loss. For clarity, the sub-themes will be briefly summarised in turn below. It should be noted, however, that in practice these sub-themes frequently overlapped.

Theme 1: health characteristics

Physical fitness

Several participants itemised the physical benefits they perceived to result from their participation in a chosen activity. For these older adults, physiological measures such as weight loss and improved cardiovascular functioning were the markers for progress and/or maintenance, allowing them to do everyday tasks with relative ease:

> For me, it's being able to run around with my grandchildren. You know, I can't see to kick a ball that well but they know that, so they'll yell: 'It's coming granddad!' And I stop it, and kick it. If I know where it is, bang! Just being able to do that, and enjoy your life. Climb the stairs and not be gasping. Being able to enjoy and embrace everything around you. (62 year old male, with age-related macular degeneration (AMD))

At the other end of the spectrum were those who described themselves as lacking physical fitness, with inactivity the primary contributing factor:

> I really don't do much at all. I'm not fit enough, and I can't see well enough. I've found my perimeters, and I don't feel I can do any more, or go any further than that. (70 year old male, with AMD)

Activity loss

Every participant lamented some form of activity loss that had resulted from his or her sight loss. With respect to physical activities, several participants explained that the 'first thing to go' was any form of ball sport participation. Other physical activities began to carry significant risks due to impaired vision or barriers created by society:

> I used to cycle a lot on the roads. I think that would now be most unwise. I might ride my bicycle on a path, but I find riding on the roads now impossible, so I've given that up. (60 year old female, with Retinitis Pigmentosa (RP))

Participants for whom the sight loss was more severe (and/or more sudden) often expressed a loss of more general physical activities related to mobility, including walking:

> I can't really do very much at all. Before, two, three, four times a week I would go – we've got a big park nearby and I would walk around the park and along the river, which is just under four miles. And I would do that several times a week. But I can't do that now, I just can't. Never mind get out into the countryside. (74 year old male, with AMD)

Comorbidities

Juggling other chronic conditions, such as circulation and joint issues, alongside sight loss also had a negative impact on a number of the participant's capacity to walk and/or move in general.

> I can't do it now, because of the neuropathy in my legs. I have no circulation left. I'm alright up to about 20 yards, but then I can't walk any further. So even going into town, I can't walk around town. (65 year old male, with Diabetic Retinopathy (DR) and retinal haemorrhage)

In contrast, many participants described using physical activity as part of their broader health care regimen, particularly to help control other chronic conditions:

> I have diabetes, so I need to keep fit and healthy and I keep my blood sugar at a really good level. And I have a check-up every six months. They're very pleased with me, because my blood sugar's been quite stable for a long time now, and it's low. And that's only because of my diet and my exercise. It controls it. And the more I do, the healthier I am. (71 year old female, with glaucoma and AMD)

Mental and emotional health

Going beyond physical health, the majority of participants acknowledged the effect of their sight loss on their mental and emotional health. Several participants recounted struggling with depression upon diagnosis, and many made an explicit link between their mental health and physical activity. For example, many explained how participation in physical activity, whether in an organised group or not, offered one the means and reason to 'get out of the house', thereby decreasing their feelings of isolation and providing a sense of purpose:

> I know that if people don't get out from the house then they've got a problem. I mean, I know myself, if I'm stuck here and I don't get out it only takes me a day or maybe a little bit more before I'm feeling quite down. And it's very true that they say exercise helps depression. It does. There's a little lane opposite me. If I walk from here and walk up that lane, I've only got to do a couple of hundred yards and I start to feel better. (66 year old male, with retinal haemorrhage)

For those who participated in solitary physical activities, these were valued for the opportunity to engage in self-reflection, contemplation and escape. Those who preferred group or team exercise cited enjoyment of the activity alongside enjoyment of the social interaction that the activity enabled.

Challenge and independence

Those participants who were keen about the activity itself reported many reasons for being so, such as personal challenge, learning or developing a physical skill, improving scores and/or winning a competitive match. For other participants, the activity was secondary to what they perceived the activity as enabling them to do:

> I'm very conscious of my independence and I want to retain that. The cycling that I do makes my legs strong, more stable. So I'm more confident in getting around without help. I like to go out on my own and get to places, and maintain my independent lifestyle. (70 year old female, with AMD)

For those who did not (or felt they could not) participate in physical activity, it was the loss of independent mobility that they most lamented.

Theme 2: accessibility and opportunity

Transport availability and cost

Experience of transport availability and cost varied by region and was most pronounced as a barrier to participation within the South West of England, where community transport and public transport links are relatively poor. Concessionary travel passes were praised, particularly within London. Participants from the Midlands had mixed experiences, depending on their proximity to urban centres and available transport links.

Variety, sustainability and consistency of opportunities

Several participants praised their local sight loss organisation for the type and variety of physical activity opportunities, and others were less pleased. Many of the latter lamented the lack of consistency of opportunity and referred to activities that were promised and then not delivered or offered and then taken away. Generally speaking, those less satisfied with available opportunities tended to be less mobile and more dependent on others. Variety of opportunity was also highly dependent on funding, which leads to important concerns being raised about the consistency and sustainability of leisure and physical activity opportunities in this context:

> Archery they started once, never heard of it again. Tandem riding – I went on one ride and I've not heard anything since. Gardening started, and then it stopped. And that's worse than not having it at all, to be honest. It raises people up, and down they come again. (70 year old female, with detached retina)

Marketing of opportunities

Several participants expressed interest in participating in organised physical activities for the visually impaired, but explained that they were unsure of what opportunities existed – and how to go about finding out about them. Those who had participated in such activities recalled having proactively and persistently sought information about available opportunities in their area.

Social support

Many participants reported not having their desired level of social support, or having lost it for various reasons – thus making their participation in physical activity more unlikely if not impossible. On the other hand, several participants described their participation in physical activity as only being possible because of the support of an individual or organisation:

> I've gone tandem cycling with the same friend – we celebrate 20 years of riding together next year. I've every confidence in him... We try to get out at least once a week, and in the summer we stop for petrol at a local pub sometimes. So that's nice – it's a real pleasure, actually. (66 year old male, with AMD)

Confidence, fear and safety

Many people felt they lacked confidence for participation in physical activity. This was often linked to a fear of injury/falling, of being out of their controlled environment. Participants expressed many additional fears: getting lost, looking silly and being a target for crime. Confidence, fear and concerns with safety had implications not just for mobility, but also for the types of physical activity that participants engaged in – and the types of activity that they could imagine themselves engaging in.

Time

The majority of participants referred to how the experience of time had changed for them. They described having to accept that everything will take them longer and as such, life had a different cadence to it – including aspects of mobility and participation in physical activities. Other participants were less accepting of the increased time that physical tasks and activities may now require. These participants bemoaned that it often took longer to get there and back than performing the activity itself.

Leisure facilities and the built and natural environment

Several participants were members of local gyms and attended regularly, reporting positive experiences. However, many of these positive stories were coupled with reports of previously poor experiences. Participants recounted being turned away because of health and safety regulations or being asked to pay more money (in addition to a membership) to have a dedicated personal trainer at every gym session. Participants' experiences (good and bad) strongly underlined that there are many considerations in making a gym facility accessible. These include accessible machinery, allocated time slots to use facilities, staff awareness and training, lighting, signage, permanence/consistency of obstacles, locker and changing rooms and a disability-friendly culture.

The built environment outside of buildings and facilities also offered many considerations, including pavement quality and grade, the location of bollards, street signs, rubbish bins and so on. Participants explained that navigating the built environment took mental as well as physical energy, and this could limit physical activity participation. Similarly, the natural environment posed many obstacles that restrict the type, level and location of physical activity engaged in by participants:

> I used to belong to a rambling group but it got to the point where I thought, no, I can't do this anymore. So I stopped. Tree roots, steps, things like that... Because I can't see the ground, I don't know if it's sloped or going up. You don't half jar your back all the time, if you aren't expecting a change in ground level. I've been whacked in the face with branches. (69 year old female, with AMD)

Reflections and conclusions

Older adults with visual impairment describe various barriers, motivating factors and facilitators to their participation in physical activity. For our participants, the interaction of these had a significant impact on physical as well as mental and emotional health. As a result, attention to this issue has important implications with respect to wellbeing and quality of life for this population.

Reported barriers to physical activity participation encompassed physical, structural and psychological realms. The barriers expressed under the broad theme of 'health characteristics' (physical fitness, activity loss, comorbidities, mental and emotional health and challenge and independence) are not necessarily exclusive to those with visual impairment. Aspects of each could easily be seen to apply generally to older adults with respect to physical activity participation, with accompanying nuances of managing visual impairment therein. It is thus critical to acknowledge that age-related sight loss does not occur in isolation, but as part of the ageing process alongside other age-related illnesses, conditions and changes. Given the growing proportion of older adults experiencing and living with sight loss, this underlines the necessity of the incorporation of visual impairment (and disability in general) into the larger 'ageing well' agenda rather than it being addressed in isolation (Jeppsson Grassman and Witaker, 2013; Raymond et al., 2014).

Many additional barriers were identified within the broad theme entitled 'accessibility and opportunity'. These barriers were more specific to individuals with visual impairment and encompassed such things as transport availability and cost; variety, sustainability and consistency of opportunities; marketing of opportunities; social support; fear, confidence and safety; time; leisure facilities; and the built and natural environment. All of these barriers are arguably amplified for older adults with visual impairment. For example, these individuals are more likely to have limited financial resources and smaller social support networks, thus further limiting engagement in leisure and physical activities. As such, those ageing with a visual impairment can be seen to be subject to a form of intersectional exclusion, on the basis of disability (sight loss specifically) and with respect to the expectations and implications of age and ageing.

Another related conclusion of this project is that each of the identified barriers has the potential (and likelihood) of overlapping and/or co-existing rather than occurring in isolation. For example, addressing the accessibility of the physical built environment within a fitness facility might need to be considered alongside the social and psychoemotional barriers that visually impaired older adults may also face. A social-relational model of disability better encapsulates the entirety and complexity of this experience – and substantiates calls for the expansion of the social model of disability (Smith and Sparkes, 2012; Thomas,

1997). For example, an impaired person's psycho-emotional wellbeing might be damaged when a group of people at the gym aim hurtful words at them or when the gym manager claims that because they are visually impaired they pose a 'health and safety' liability. In such social interactions, the potential damage and/or undermining of the visually impaired older adult's psycho-emotional wellbeing might result in their future avoidance of the gym altogether. Hence, damage to psycho-emotional wellbeing can place limits on what one can do and can become. Attention to the sociology of impairment with emphasis on lived experience, and phenomenology in particular, holds much promise for future work in this area (Hughes and Paterson, 1997; Paterson and Hughes, 1999).

With respect to motivating factors for participation in physical activity, older adults with visual impairment described many perceived physical benefits such as improved physical fitness, help in controlling other health conditions and implications for independence and mobility. In addition, many active participants also cited the mental and emotional rewards of participation. Engaging in activities often also offered the opportunity for social interaction, and this brought immense pleasure. Awareness of the variety of motivators for participation in physical activity has the potential to inform in public health messages and/or promotion within this population. For example, in addition to highlighting the health benefits of participation, it may be fruitful to emphasise the implications of these health benefits. Across the board, independence was valued by older adults with sight loss. Making clearer links between participation in physical activity and maintaining independence has the potential to increase action and participation (that is, improved balance, decreased incidence of falls, fewer reports of mental health issues, etc.). Going one step further, health promotion messages would do well to highlight the social benefits of participation in physical activity and to underscore the potential for pleasure and social engagement within such activities.

Including visually impaired older adults who considered themselves to be physically active within our sample allowed an exploration of the facilitators of their involvement. These included such things as social support, access to and information about desirable activities, confidence and accessible transportation enabling their participation. Once again, these facilitators overlap and are important to consider in their interactions rather than individually. However, individual stories about facilitators are excellent examples of what has worked well for some, could work well for others – and provide a starting point for an examination of promising practice. For example, when designing/conceptualising a physical activity opportunity specifically for older adults with visual impairment, it is most important to ask older adults with visual impairment what *they* want. Subsequent targeted marketing of the opportunity will lead to increased engagement and could limit the 'start/stop' nature of many activity programmes. Further, there is a demonstrated need for all service providers to examine their inclusivity practices and address inclusion as a whole, including accessible facilities, equipment, staff-training, marketing and development. It is important that these components are addressed both within and beyond the realm of fitness facilities to encompass other physical activity settings and opportunities.

Currently, many local sight loss organisations, ageing charities and physical activity providers offer a 'one size fits all' social activity group, thus fulfilling directives and/or requirements to address the social and leisure needs of older adults with visual impairment. However, there is a danger of a tick-box approach here. No one social group can satisfy the needs and desires of a heterogeneous population. For many participants of this project, existing social activity groups were insufficient and/or too inactive to suit their leisure and activity purposes and preferences. Critical attention to the above points would ensure a range of available opportunities, wherever possible. That said, all of the above is a large request of resource-restricted, often non-profit, local sight loss organisations. There is a need to work collaboratively with national sight loss organisations (and crucially, national ageing organisations) to pool resources and knowledge and to ensure development and consistency of opportunity across the country. It is also necessary to engage community and commercial stakeholders in the matter of inclusion and to widen accessibility and promote compliance to anti-discrimination laws. Only then can the notion of ageing well (through physicality) be a truly viable option for older adults with late onset sight loss.

Acknowledgements

This research was undertaken when the author was an Associate Research Fellow based at the European Centre for the Environment and Health (ECEHH – part of the University of Exeter Medical School), which is part financed by the European Regional Development Fund Programme 2007 to 2013 and European Social Fund Convergence Programme for Cornwall and the Isles of Scilly. This was a collaborative project between ECEHH (Drs. Cassandra Phoenix, Meridith Griffin) and the Peter Harrison Centre for Disability Sport at Loughborough University (Drs.

Brett Smith, P. David Howe) and was funded by the Thomas Pocklington Trust, a sight loss charity in the United Kingdom. The content does not necessarily represent the official views of the funding organisation.

References

Braun V and Clark V (2006) Using thematic analysis in psychology. *Qualitative Research in Psychology* 3: 77–101.

Craig R, Mindell J and Hirani V (2008) *Health Survey for England 2008: Physical Activity and Fitness*. Volume 1. London: NHS Information for Health and Social Care.

Crews JE and Campbell VA (2001) Health conditions, activity limitations, and participation restrictions among older people with visual impairments. *Journal of Visual Impairment and Blindness* 95: 453–467.

Department of Health (DoH) (2013) Improving quality of life for people with long term conditions. Available at: https://www.gov.uk/government/policies/improving-quality-of-life-for-people-with-long-term-conditions (accessed September 2013).

Department for Work and Pensions (DWP) (2013) Fulfilling potential: building a deeper understanding of disability in the UK today. Available at: http://odi.dwp.gov.uk/fulfilling-potential/index.php (accessed January 2013).

English Longitudinal Study of Ageing (ELSA) (2013) Available at: http://www.elsa-project.ac.uk/ (accessed January 2013). Full datasets available at: http://discover.ukdataservice.ac.uk/catalogue?sn=5050

Fight for Sight (2013) Statistics about blindness and eye disease. Available at: http://www.fightforsight.org.uk/statistics-about-blindness-and-eye-disease (accessed January 2013).

Freund P (2001) Bodies, disability and spaces: the social model and disabling spatial organisations. *Disability and Society* 16(5): 689–706.

Goodley D (2011) *Disability Studies*. London: Sage.

Green J and Thorogood N (2009) *Qualitative Research Methods for Health Care* (2nd edition). London: Sage.

Hughes B and Paterson K (1997) The social model of disability and the disappearing body: towards a sociology of impairment. *Disability and Society* 12(3): 325–340.

Jeppsson Grassman E and Witaker A (2013) *Ageing with Disability: A Lifecourse Perspective*. Bristol: Policy Press.

Jones GC, Rovner BW, Crews JE et al. (2009). Effects of depressive symptoms on health behaviour practices among older adults with vision loss. *Rehabilitation Psychology* 54(2): 164–172.

Kennedy J and Minkler M (1998) Disability theory and public policy: implications for critical gerontology. *International Journal of Health Services* 28(4): 757–776.

Paterson K and Hughes B (1999) Disability studies and phenomenology: the carnal politics of everyday life. *Disability and Society* 14(5): 597–610.

Priestly M (2003) *Disability: A Life Course Approach*. Cambridge: Polity Press.

Priestly M and Rabiee P (2002) Same difference? older people's organisations and disability issues. *Disability and Society* 17(6): 597–611.

Raymond E, Grenier A and Hanley J (2014) Community participation of older adults with disabilities. *Journal of Community and Applied Social Psychology* 24(1): 50–62.

Smith B and Sparkes AC (2012) Disability, sport and physical activity: a critical review. In: N Watson, A Roulstone and C Thomas (eds) *Routledge Handbook of Disability Studies*. London: Routledge, pp. 336–347.

Sparkes AC and Smith B (2014) *Qualitative Research Methods in Sport, Exercise and Health*. London: Routledge.

Sport England (2011) Active people survey 5: disability trends and barriers. Available at: http://www.sportengland.org/research/active_people_survey/aps5.aspx?sortBy=alpha&pageNum=1 (accessed January 2013).

Sport England (2013) Active people survey 7: once a week participation in sport. Available at: http://www.sportengland.org/media/162187/01_1x30_overall_factsheet_aps7q2-final.pdf (accessed August 2013).

Thomas C (2007) *Sociologies of Disability and Illness*. London: Palgrave.

Townsend P (2007) Using human rights to defeat ageism: dealing with policy-induced 'structured dependency'. In: M Bernard and T Scharf (eds) *Critical Perspectives on Ageing Societies*. Bristol: Policy Press, pp. 27–44.

Tulle E (2008) Acting your age? sports science and the ageing body. *Journal of Aging Studies* 22(4): 340–347.

16
Local Environments and Activity in Later Life: Meaningful Experiences in Green and Blue Spaces

Sarah L. Bell and Benedict W. Wheeler

Populations across much of the world are ageing. In the UK, 1 in 5 people will be aged 65 and over by 2020 (Allen, 2008). This has sparked growing interest in the potential to develop 'healthy communities which support older people to live lives which are as fulfilling as possible' (Department of Health, 2001: 107). Such interest is based on the recognition that, contrary to existing narratives of decline, 'old age can also be marked by the acquisition of new roles and, potentially, be a flourishing time of mobility and new creativity' (Gilroy, 2012: 74–75).

In this chapter, we focus on the role of place characteristics in promoting physical activity in older age. Specifically, we consider 'green space' (urban parks, countryside, woodlands, gardens etc.) and 'blue space' (coast, riverside, lakes and urban waterways). Past studies have suggested that green spaces can provide older adults with appealing spaces for gentle physical activity (Sugiyama and Ward Thompson, 2008), social interaction (Kweon et al., 1998), restoration and recovery from stress or fatigue (Berto, 2007) and the forging of new social identities (Milligan et al., 2005). Different types of green and blue space interaction may enable people to engage in positive meaningful experiences whilst negotiating the changes associated with ageing. Such efforts often inherently involve physical activity, even if it is not the primary motivation for engaging with these spaces. For example, the desire to spend meaningful time with the family may lead to enhanced physical activity whilst playing with grandchildren in the park or at the beach.

The chapter starts with a brief review of the literature examining the benefits of engaging with green and blue spaces in older age. This is followed by an exploration of these benefits in the context of both individual and shared green and blue space experiences, drawing on the novel findings of an in-depth interpretive study conducted in two towns in south west England.

The benefits of active engagement in green and blue space in later life

Older age is associated with periods of significant change, including shifts linked to retirement, personal and spousal health, caring duties and bereavement (Parry et al., 2004). These changes have both negative and positive impacts on the daily lives of older adults; whilst the end of paid employment may allow time for engagement in new or long-standing interests and family commitments, the associated loss of income and declines in mobility can create new difficulties (Gilroy, 2008). The diverse configurations of these changes and the varying capacity of older adults to adapt to them renders this a highly heterogeneous group, 'encompassing two or three generations, a spectrum of faiths and a diversity of wealth and income levels and cut across by gender, sexuality, disability, "race" and ethnicity' (Gilroy, 2008: 149).

Studies exploring the use of green and blue spaces in later life suggest a potential role for these spaces in promoting opportunities for physical activity amongst those who choose to do so. For example, 2 research programmes in the UK – I'DGO ('Inclusive Design for Getting Outdoors') and I'DGO too[1] – have explored how local environments (specifically those within and around green open spaces) could be designed more inclusively to meet the mobility needs of older adults in order to enhance their sense of competence and improve their quality of life. This work suggested that recreational walking can be encouraged through proximity to 'pleasant' open spaces (defined as those with a welcoming and relaxing atmosphere, well-maintained trees and plants and opportunities for children's play and positive social interaction) and a lack of antisocial or 'nuisance' behaviour. Walking for transport was influenced by the perceived presence of 'good' facilities (including toilets, seating, shelters and inclusive activities) and 'good' paths en route to the open space (enjoyable paths considered easy to walk along, with no perceived obstacles) (Sugiyama and Ward Thompson, 2008; Alves et al., 2008).

The value of being able to walk to local green spaces has been identified in other studies, with parks noted as one of several 'third places' contributing to older adults' 'natural neighbourhood networks' (Gardner, 2011). These places are characterised as accessible, socially inclusive, a 'home from home', and conducive to unplanned social interaction and easy, impromptu conversation with other visitors. Gardner notes how such chance encounters offered participants a 'nourished sense of self, companionship, a sense of purpose, and a more positive outlook on life' (2011: 267). This was also apparent within Chow's (2013) interview-based study of older adult park users in Taiwan in which participants appreciated the fitness equipment in their local parks as a focal point for social interaction. Notably, few participants visited the park specifically to use the outdoor fitness equipment, but many used it once there due to the social setting of the equipment area. As one participant commented: 'you come here frequently and you become familiar with the other people here, then you become friends' (2013: 1221).

Other studies have identified the value of park spaces for older adults in promoting opportunities for meaningful family interaction and intergenerational play. For example, Spencer et al. (2013) conducted a series of focus groups to explore the possible contribution of public open spaces to play amongst older people living in Bristol, UK. Participants described the pleasure of 'joining in the fun' when playing with grandchildren or when watching other people acting playfully. Interestingly, participants suggested they needed an 'excuse' to play in such spaces, be it the presence of grandchildren, inclusive age-appropriate outdoor gym equipment, walking trails marked with suggested activities or taking part in organised events such as celebrations and festivals. Importantly, feelings of safety and comfort were noted as prerequisites for such playful attitudes and pursuits. Linked to this, intergenerational tensions and perceived antisocial behaviour have been noted as significant barriers to active green space engagement amongst older adults (O'Brien, 2006; Seamen et al., 2010).

In-depth qualitative studies have highlighted the potential for green spaces to promote other types of pleasurable (often active) experiences in later life. For example, Milligan et al. (2004) discuss older adults' enjoyment of the natural environment when engaging in new hobbies, such as painting, photography and walking. These adults described certain urban built landscapes as 'depressing' or 'threatening at times' and therefore greatly appreciated the chance to 'step out' and enjoy the peace and tranquillity of nature. The garden, in particular, was valued as a site of mental and physical renewal, with references made to restorative multisensory encounters within such spaces (e.g. pausing to appreciate birds singing and flower scents and colours).

The sense of creativity and achievement gained through working in the garden was also noted as important by the older communal gardeners in Milligan et al.'s (2004) study. This is mirrored in the accounts of older adults engaged in environmental volunteering initiatives. For example, Townsend (2006) reports on a series of projects undertaken by the NiCHE (Nature, Community, Health and Environment) research group at Deakin University, Australia. These projects illustrate that participation in a group involved in voluntary conservation activities exposes people to the restorative benefits of the natural environment, the social benefits of meeting other people and opportunities to make a contribution that is socially valued. Older participants, in particular, commented on their sense of achievement, pride and ownership of the work they had undertaken and the benefits of enhanced community involvement and improved social networks.

The social benefits of communal gardening and environmental volunteering initiatives appear to extend beyond the activities themselves. For example, participants in a qualitative study of members of a community garden in Melbourne, Australia, highlighted its value as 'a supportive and an easy place to discuss issues going on in their lives', including deep personal issues such as illness or bereavement (Kingsley et al., 2009: 212). Reflecting on the findings of their qualitative study with older gardeners in Carlisle, Milligan et al. (2005: 60) highlight the role of the communal garden in supporting 'the forging of new social identities within new social networks, providing spaces in which it is possible to drop the "mask of ageing", and allowing older people to shift away from their socially prescribed roles'. They describe the communal garden as a 'home from home' without the complexities or burdens of domestic familial relationships.

However, these studies have also discussed the limitations posed by advancing age on older adults' capacity to cope with the garden or to continue participating in social or community activities as they used to (Milligan et al., 2004). These changes may lead to distress, frustration or even depression, particularly amongst those who initially became involved in an effort to bring routine and purpose to their retirement (Gross and Lane, 2007). Research suggests that agentic 'preparation' or 'coping' practices may help to deal with these shifts. Examples from a gardening perspective include the gradual replacement of labour-intensive aspects of the garden (such as vegetables and shrubs) with tubs, hanging baskets, lawned or paved areas, as well as participating in communal gardening schemes where individuals maintain each other's gardens in the event of illness or short holiday periods (Milligan et al.,

2004). These are examples of 'adaptive optimising strategies' (Wiles et al., 2009: 665), whereby individuals shift their actions to maximise opportunities to experience preferred green spaces in the face of new constraints emerging within their everyday lives.

Older adults' active green space use within two urban areas in Cornwall, UK

This section draws on the findings of a study exploring the complex personal and structural factors that define and drive individual choices regarding the use of different green and blue spaces over time. More specifically, it examines how participants' interactions with these places were shaped by their personal life circumstances, their local environment and their past place experiences.

As detailed by Bell et al. (2015), an interpretive, mixed methods 'geo-narrative' approach was designed for the study, with a purposive sample of 33 participants recruited from two towns in Cornwall, south west England. Participants carried an accelerometer (measuring physical activity) and Global Positioning System (GPS, measuring location) receiver for 1 week. The resulting data were used to produce personalised activity maps, showing where participants went that week, how long they stayed in different places and how active they were. Each participant's maps were then used as visual prompts to guide an in-depth interview exploring how and why they engage with different local environments to promote and maintain a sense of wellbeing. This was followed by a series of case study go-along interviews for a subset of participants, in places they deemed important, offering further insights into the lived experiences and relationships playing out within such places. In order to gain insights into the value of green and blue spaces for wellbeing across a diversity of everyday situations, the full study sample captured variation in gender, life circumstances and green/blue space engagement. In this chapter, we focus on insights gained from 9 retired participants, focusing in particular on the experiences discussed by 5 participants: Evelyn, Bill, Grace, Linda and Ron.

First, we introduce Evelyn, who took part in the pilot study; Evelyn moved to Cornwall from Yorkshire with her husband over 20 years ago and had taken early retirement a couple of years prior to participating in the study. During the interview, she explained that she used to do aerobics and run the equivalent of half marathons once or twice a week but had injured her back a few years ago and had therefore switched to more gentle activities, including yoga, pilates and dog walking. As indicated below, certain green/blue space walking routes were particularly important to her as they felt safe and familiar due to time spent there as a family in the past. This helped her to control her anxiety when walking the dog alone. Importantly, this anxiety was not directly linked to her personal safety, but to a concern that she would not know what to do should they meet a particularly aggressive dog. Through walking in places where she felt at ease, she was able to enjoy and completely immerse herself in the walks:

> Sarah: Ok, so here we have a coastal visit I think?
>
> Evelyn: ...Mm I played on the beach [with the dog] for a little bit, and then walked up the valley at the back. Normally I'd walk up here and then up to the top here [pointing inland on the map] and you can circle all the way down over the cliffs and back down again...but on that day, it was an absolutely horrible day and we just walked up here and back again...
>
> Sarah: What do you tend to be thinking about whilst you're walking the dog?
>
> Evelyn: Um [pause] I wouldn't say that I necessarily think about anything other than where I am and what I'm looking at. I think I would more concentrate on 'ooh that's a really nice flower' or 'the stream's very full today' or whatever...
>
> Sarah: Ah ok and is there anything else that draws you to that particular area?
>
> Evelyn: Um when the kids were small we used to love going there rather than [the next] beach because that was so big and full of people whereas here [points to the beach on the map] was always a bit [quieter]. And it was my mum's favourite beach actually so that might be partly why we used to go there a lot...it just feels comfortable.

Second, we introduce Bill; Bill moved to Cornwall from London with his wife in his early 40s, where they started a family and both underwent significant career changes. Bill later phased in his retirement over 3 years and now values the extra time he has to engage in both existing and new hobbies. His allotment, in particular, emerged as an important space, in part for providing appealing opportunities for physical activity, but also through acting as one of several outdoor open areas where he feels calm and relaxed. He noted a 'natural affinity' and positive 'emotional response' towards such spaces. When asked why he initially decided to get an allotment, Bill explained that he used to dread going to the gym and perceived the allotment to be a more enjoyable (and less expensive) source of physical activity, contributing to his long-term fitness and providing opportunities for satisfying, short-term cathartic

Green and Blue Spaces 181

release ('heaving things around') within a more pleasurable environment than that experienced in the gym. Such comments illustrate that, for participants like Bill, engaging in their preferred activity was about both the physicality of it *and* the sensual and emotional benefits of being outdoors (Cosgriff et al., 2009; Krenichyn, 2006):

> **Bill:** *(when asked why he decided to get an allotment):* Ten years ago I started going to the gym because I was kind of physically inactive and I was putting on weight. I was physically weak, my body strength just wasn't good, and I suddenly realised that I really needed to do something about it. So I went to the gym for a few years and then I thought well, I hate going to the gym, it's like, it's a chore, you know – 'oh God it's the gym again today' – so I thought, well I need to do something that keeps me physically active, gets me outdoors, and then when I finish work I can go there, heave things around and do stuff. So really, that was it [the decision to start an allotment], it was about physical activity and being outdoors...and, you know, the allotment costs £2 a week, and the gym was costing me twelve or something!

Other study participants noted their enjoyment simply of being outdoors in nature; although they walked within these spaces, the primary motivation was to connect to nature rather than being physically active. This was most apparent in the accounts of Grace, a participant in her 70s who moved to Cornwall with her husband (who has now passed away) in their retirement nearly 20 years ago. Grace explained that she had always 'escaped' into nature, even as a child. During the interview, she discussed her appreciation of a wooded path behind her house. The path eventually meets a nature reserve and opens up to Swanpool (a brackish lagoon supporting a variety of wildlife species and a neighbouring beach), which she visited whilst wearing the GPS and accelerometer. This is discussed in the interview extract below:

> **Sarah:** *Can you tell me about the Swanpool trip?*
> **Grace:** *It's lovely to walk, I mean if it had been a lovely week of weather I would've walked far more along the [sea] front...through the woods, by the stream, it's beautiful in there...*
> **Sarah:** *What is it about Swanpool that draws you?*
> **Grace:** *Well it's just our nearest beach and I love to see the wildlife on the pool. It's rather unusual isn't it? I think it's the third largest natural pool in the country, something like that. You see a lot of birds, especially in the winter. They all fly in, all the little tufted ducks, whilst over the summer it's quite deserted.*

Later in the interview, when asked about the woods leading down to Swanpool, Grace explained her appreciation of engaging with nature's seasonal cycles and the peace afforded by such areas (though notes that noisy dogs can compromise the experience). Interestingly, whilst she used to enjoy more remote coastal and countryside walks, she has become more wary of these areas since her husband passed away and with older age, for both personal safety and mobility reasons:

> **Sarah:** *And what do you tend to notice when you're walking along the wooded path?*
> **Grace:** *Hopefully quiet and not too many dogs barking. Much as I like dogs, they do make an awful racket in the woods. I just like everything. The trees, and you notice how things are growing and changing, just peaceful.*
> **Sarah:** *Can you describe any other local walks that you like?*
> **Grace:** *Umm [sighs] I suppose I tend not to walk as much as I used to. I mean I'd think nothing of five or ten miles years ago but not now [smiles]...I mean places that I really, really like that are lonely and quiet, but I would avoid those now...you never quite know what's going to [hesitates] I'd be careful in the lonely places.*

For other participants, physical activity often coincided with meaningful time spent with the extended family. This was particularly apparent during Linda's interview. Linda was in her early 60s and in the process of shifting from partial to full retirement. She had lived in Cornwall ever since moving there with her parents during her mid-teens. Much of Linda's physical activity occurred through quality time spent with her husband and with the wider family (particularly her grandson), highlighting the importance of shared active experiences. Linda valued local woodland, coastal and countryside trails where she walks with her husband and daughter, whilst her grandson cycles safely along beside them. When asked what makes a 'good' walk, she noted several local examples, in each case highlighting the importance of the natural elements of the space, together with practical facilities such as car parking and opportunities to stop for an ice cream or picnic:

> **Linda** *(whilst explaining what makes a 'good' walk locally):* We like to sort of walk somewhere and then do something and then come back again...another walk that we sometimes do is up over Carn Grey at the top. The china clay [industry] have made trails around so you can walk round them quite easily, and again parking is so, so important – you've got to be able to park, you know free parking – and there's two free spots up there where we can park. Um so yes having a walk round there's nice 'cos you can walk round the pits and the water's in the pit, and our grandson can take his bike

> *and cycle around. We just stroll along, and then we go blackberry-picking up the top there as well which is really nice. I think the views as well, you know, having a nice view, being able to see open spaces and countryside – that I find enjoyable"*

The efforts made by participants to maximise opportunities for positive shared experiences were particularly apparent within the accounts of the oldest participant in the study, Ron. Now in their 80s and 70s, respectively, Ron and his wife Olive have lived and worked together in and around the study area for most of their lives. Throughout the interviews, they tended to answer together, with their activities reflecting their preferences and needs as a couple (including Olive's love of wildlife and Ron's health needs after having a heart attack and gastrectomy). As indicated in the interview extract below, they discussed Ron's difficulties in navigating places with hills, and the importance of places with cafes so that he can eat small but regular meals. This has ruled out some of their favourite inland and coastal walks, such that they tend to visit more navigable green spaces like the Eden Project, the Lost Gardens of Heligan (both local horticultural attractions) or Par Beach (a flat, easily accessible local beach):

> **Sarah:** *How if at all did the GPS and accelerometer influence you that week?*
> **Ron:** *Well, we hadn't been to Heligan for perhaps a fortnight ... any free afternoon, if we don't know what else to do, we might go down there.*
> **Olive:** *We tend to go there more than Eden don't we?*
> **Sarah:** *Why is that?*
> **Olive:** *Umm, accessibility for a start, umm Eden's fine but getting down there always isn't easy is it?*
> **Ron:** *Yeah, wherever you park at Eden, you may be able to get a bus, you know, back to the car park but there's a fair slope to walk up to where the bus takes you from, so um that would possibly influence that yes.*
> **Olive:** *Whereas down at Heligan you park on the level, and*
> **Ron:** *And you walk on the level.*
> **Olive:** *And you walk on the level and I mean we don't go down to the jungle down there because that's too much of climb for him, we used to didn't we but latterly we haven't done it.*
> **Ron:** *So [pause] trying to keep things on a level keel [laughs] is what I would explain our differences now from ten years ago. We would be more adventurous then in going to places with steeper slopes ...*
> **Olive:** *Well since you've had your heart attack you can't do it can you?*
> **Ron:** *Well, it's not wise.*

The challenge posed by even shallow inclines was particularly apparent during their go-along interview, where Ron was unable to walk along some of the paths that were theoretically 'accessible'. Whilst the location had been designed to include features that would lessen structural barriers to use and maximise accessibility, it was clear during the go-along interview that these efforts were primarily aimed at wheelchair users. As Ron noted, even the provision of additional, regular seating opportunities could enhance his use of the space. This example highlights the need to understand the importance placed by older adults on both individual and shared place experiences. Prioritising the latter, Ron and Olive were adapting their activities and place interactions together to accommodate Ron's health and mobility needs. In doing so, previously valued active interactions with more 'natural' green and blue spaces have been replaced by green spaces that are easier to negotiate, such as their own and public gardens and accessible beaches.

Conclusions

With a growing number of people living longer in the UK and further afield, supporting and nurturing positive active experiences in later life are key aspects of maintaining population health. This chapter has examined the use of local natural environments, specifically green and blue spaces, for meaningful active ageing. In doing so, it has emphasised the need to recognise the wider motivations that might be driving active place interactions in older age.

Given the heterogeneous nature of the older population, it is important to recognise that older adults may approach physical activity in diverse ways. Some may be driven primarily by health concerns, a passion for a particular sport or physical activity, or a need for a sense of purpose, achievement and/or creativity in older age. The latter is commonly noted as a key benefit of personal and communal garden spaces (Gross and Lane, 2007; Milligan et al., 2004). As discussed in the second half of this chapter, other individuals may be more motivated by opportunities to spend time in a place they value. In the context of the study findings presented here, these included open spaces (e.g. Bill's emotional or 'natural affinity' for open spaces like his allotment) and places encouraging feelings of connection to nature (e.g. Grace's tendency to 'escape' into nature, including her local woodland walk and nature reserve where she can immerse herself in the local wildlife and appreciate nature's seasonal cycles).

Importantly, the chapter also discussed the shared nature of some of these experiences, with several participants tailoring their active place interactions to promote opportunities to spend time with significant others. For example, Linda noted the importance of being with the extended family, which often involved walking along local countryside, woodland and coastal trails with her husband, daughter and grandson. Now in the later stages of old age, Ron and Olive discussed the difficulties in negotiating these types of trails (especially since Ron's heart attack), instead valuing opportunities to wander around local horticultural attractions and accessible beaches together (prioritising places 'on the level' and with facilities).

Taken together, these findings suggest the potential for green and blue spaces to contribute to feelings of fulfilment in older age through providing opportunities for individual or shared active experiences. However, the examples provided also indicate that such place encounters may act as reminders of increased bodily vulnerability in older age. This may be in terms of the difficulties encountered in navigating previously taken-for-granted spaces or the reluctance to explore new places alone in the face of changes in personal mobility and energy levels. This underlines the importance of designing supportive, inclusive local environments (including green, blue and connecting built spaces) in which older adults can feel at ease whilst engaging in personally meaningful experiences, be it alone or with significant others.

Note

1. http://www.idgo.ac.uk/

References

Allen J (2008) *Older People and Wellbeing*. London: Institute for Public Policy Research.

Alves S, Aspinall P, Ward Thompson C and Sugiyama T (2008) Preferences of older people for environmental attributes of local parks: the use of conjoint analysis. *Facilities* 26: 433–453.

Bell SL, Phoenix C, Lovell R and Wheeler BW (2015) Using GPS and geo-narratives: a methodological approach for understanding and situating everyday green space encounters. *Area* 47: 88–96.

Berto R (2007) Assessing the restorative value of the environment: a study on the elderly in comparison with young adults and adolescents. *International Journal of Psychology* 42: 331–341.

Chow H (2013) Outdoor fitness equipment in parks: a qualitative study from older adults' perceptions. *BMC Public Health* 13: 1216–1225.

Cosgriff M, Little D and Wilson E (2009) The nature of nature: how New Zealand women in middle to later life experience nature-based leisure. *Leisure Sciences* 32: 15–32.

Department of Health (2001) *National Service Framework: For Older People*. London: HMSO.
Gardner P (2011) Natural neighbourhood networks: important social networks in the lives of older adults aging in place. *Journal of Aging Studies* 25: 263–271.
Gilroy R (2008) Places that support human flourishing: lessons from later life. *Planning Theory and Practice* 9: 145–163.
Gilroy R (2012) Wellbeing and the neighbourhood: promoting choice and independence for all ages. In: S Atkinson, S Fuller and J Painter (eds) *Wellbeing and Place*. Farnham, UK: Ashgate Publishing Limited.
Gross H and Lane N (2007) Landscapes of the lifespan: exploring accounts of own gardens and gardening. *Journal of Environmental Psychology* 27: 225–241.
Kingsley J, Townsend M and Henderson-Wilson C (2009) Cultivating health and wellbeing: members' perceptions of the health benefits of a Port Melbourne community garden. *Leisure Studies* 28: 207–219.
Krenichyn K (2006) 'The only place to go and be in the city': women talk about exercise, being outdoors, and the meanings of a large urban park. *Health and Place* 12: 631–643.
Kweon B, Sullivan W and Wiley A (1998) Green common spaces and the social interaction of inner-city older adults. *Environment and Behavior* 30: 832–858.
Milligan C, Bingley A and Gatrell A (2005) 'Healing and feeling': the place of emotions in later life. In: J Davidson, L Bondi and M Smith (eds) *Emotional Geographies*. Aldershot, UK: Ashgate.
Milligan C, Gatrell A and Bingley A (2004) 'Cultivating health': therapeutic landscapes and older people in northern England. *Social Science and Medicine* 58: 1781–1793.
O'Brien E (2006) Social housing and green space: a case study in Inner London. *Forestry* 79: 535–551.
Parry J, Vegeris S, Hudson MHB and Taylor R (2004) Independent living in later life. London: A report of research carried out by the Policy Studies Institute on behalf of the Department for Work and Pensions.
Seaman P, Jones R and Ellaway A (2010) It's not just about the park, it's about integration too: why people choose to use or not use urban green spaces. *International Journal of Behavioral Nutrition and Physical Activity* 7: 78–87.
Spencer B, Williams K, Mahdjoubi L and Sara R (2013) Third places for the third age: the contribution of playable space to the well-being of older people. In: R Coles and Z Millman (eds) *Landscape, Well-Being and Environment*. Abingdon, UK: Routledge.
Sugiyama T and Ward Thompson C (2008) Associations between characteristics of neighbourhood open space and older people's walking. *Urban Forestry and Urban Greening* 7: 41–51.
Townsend M (2006) Feel blue? Touch green! participation in forest/woodland management as a treatment for depression. *Urban Forestry and Urban Greening* 5: 111–120.
Wiles J, Allen R, Palmer A, Hayman K, Keeling S and Kerse N (2009) Older people and their social spaces: a study of well-being and attachment to place in Aotearoa New Zealand. *Social Sciences and Medicine* 68: 664–671.

Index

active ageing, 21, 32, 51, 54, 63, 65
activities, sport/physical, 56
age, third, 3, 36, 55, 101
ageing body, 2, 7, 24, 44, 72, 93, 101, 107, 113, 143
ageing women, 149
agency, 10, 18, 117, 146
Archer, 13, 18
assemblages, 106, 129, 142, 146

behaviours
  health-appropriate, 13
  health-related, 11, 76
  health-relevant, 80
bloomers, late, 54
blue spaces, 175
bodies
  active, 108
  active ageing, 102
  athletic, 10, 28, 56, 141
  communicative, 146
  decaying, 152
  disciplined, 134, 144, 146
  docile, 10
  female, 59
  fit, 9, 60
  frail, 96
  healthy, 132, 149
  lived, 116, 128
  masculine, 147
  postmodern, 35
  regulated, 34
body techniques, 46, 129
Bourdieu, 69, 79, 122, 128, 153, 159

capital, 75, 129, 153
career, 5, 45, 67
care settings, 5, 81
chronic conditions, 54, 133, 166
class, 2, 56, 69, 84, 113
communities, 40, 82, 106, 172
consumption, 2, 26, 36, 55, 125
continuers, 54

counter-narratives, 146
counterstories, 96, 107
countryside, 105, 165, 175
cultural practices, 44

dance, 85
dementia, 63, 93, 161
dependency, 3, 26, 55, 107, 113
depression, 49, 82, 166, 178
diabetes, 43
disability, 14, 39, 65, 78, 161, 170, 176
discourses
  contemporary public health, 132
  neo-liberal health, 125
dispositions, 3, 58, 69, 145
Durkheim, 129, 135

embodied identities, 39
embodied intoxication–, 134
embodied practices, 32, 38, 51, 127
embodiment, 2, 11, 56, 104, 111, 112, 124, 142
environment, natural, 169, 177
exercise
  leisure-oriented, 48
  stretching, 28
exercise adherence, 117
exercise and health, 36
exercise practices, 119, 120
exercise prescriptions, 113
exercise science, 70, 113
existential capital, 124, 129

families, aspiring middle class, 78
family cultures, 75
Featherstone, 36
femininities, 143
fitness, pursuit of, 35, 60, 125
floorball, 151
football, 61, 75, 149, 150
Foucault, 10, 20, 40, 153
Fourth Age, 55
frailty, 2, 24, 55, 93, 147

geo-narratives, 8, 109, 179
Goffman, 23, 30
grandparents, 71
green spaces, 175
gym, 82, 137, 171, 180

habitus, 69, 70, 115, 128, 144
 narrative, 145
health
 emotional, 166, 170
 good, 16, 46, 119
 ill, 65, 78, 107, 114
 imperative of, 39
 will to, 34, 125
health behaviours, 105, 121, 133
health benefits, 70, 73, 109, 154, 171
health discourses, 70, 154
healthism, 152
health policy, 34, 109
health problems, 48, 133, 149
health professionals, 51, 109, 124
health promotion, 34, 66, 117
healthy ageing, 36

identity, 23, 40, 58, 104, 128, 137
illness, chronic, 44, 109
illness trajectory, 46
inactivity, 2, 15, 37, 63, 165
independence, 27, 85, 146, 161, 171
interventions, 3, 8, 10, 16, 17, 93, 109, 150
intoxication, embodied, 129

jogging, 33, 116, 151

Katz, 13, 22, 101

landscape, 129, 142, 177
lifestories, 93
lifestyles, 13, 23, 39, 45, 81, 115
 health-related, 16
lived experiences, 22, 70, 145, 162, 179

masculinities, 32, 76, 131, 137, 143
master athletes, 36, 72
Masters Sport, 10, 55
modernity, 39, 55, 101, 117
muscles, 27, 46, 63, 76, 126, 139, 156

narrative, 9, 37, 85, 92, 93, 138, 146
narrative, of decline, 70, 88, 101, 102, 147
narrative foreclosure, 94
neoliberal societies, 21

PA, family cultures of, 75
pains, embodied, 130
patients, 46
physical activity participation, 2, 169
physical activity, pleasures of, 35, 101, 102, 114, 116, 130, 171
physical capital, 128, 141, 153
physical culture practices, 116
physical exercise, regular, 43
pleasure, typology of, 102
power, 10, 18, 20, 37, 107, 139, 152
public health, 5, 13, 32, 117, 124

rekindlers, 54
residential care, 81, 84
resistance, 9, 54, 72, 83, 95, 107
retirement, 21, 37, 44, 81, 105, 176
risk, 22, 33, 43, 54, 88, 94, 114, 165

SB (sedentary behaviour), 9, 11
self-care, 50, 55, 120
sight loss, 161
sitting, 11, 14, 23, 25, 63, 64, 75
social model, 8
society, somatic, 34
spaces, 7, 105, 120, 125, 139, 141, 143, 155, 175
sport commitment, 80
sport continuers, 57
sport participation, 60
sport performance, 144
sport psychology, 117
sports career, 141
sport science, 4, 10
stillness, 95, 121, 139
storyteller, 93, 99
subcultures, sporting, 145
successful ageing, 21, 102, 113
sweating, 119, 150
swimmers, 26

team sports, 7, 158, 159
tennis, 57–58
therapeutic education, 44
training, 10, 56, 145, 157, 169
Turner, 33

visual impairment, 161, 163, 164, 169, 170, 171, 172

Wacquant, 127, 128
well-being, 8, 33, 83, 88, 107
wisdom, ordinary, 93

youthism, 152

Zygmunt Bauman, 34

Printed and bound by CPI Group (UK) Ltd, Croydon, CR0 4YY